COMMONSENSE USE OF MEDICINES

COMMONSENSE USE OF MEDICINES

John Fry
General Practitioner, Beckenham, Kent

John Trounce
Emeritus Professor of Clinical Pharmacology and Physician at Guy's Hospital, London

Martin Godfrey
Medical Editor, *MIMS Magazine*, London

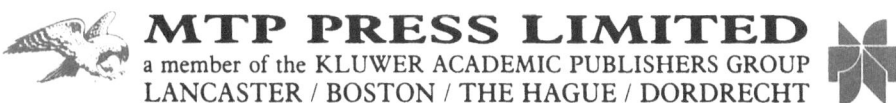

MTP PRESS LIMITED
a member of the KLUWER ACADEMIC PUBLISHERS GROUP
LANCASTER / BOSTON / THE HAGUE / DORDRECHT

Published in the UK and Europe by
MTP Press Limited
Falcon House
Lancaster, England

British Library Cataloguing in Publication Data

Fry, John, *1922–*
    Commonsense use of medicines.—
    (Commonsense series).
    1. Drugs—Prescribing
    I. Title   II. Trounce, J.R.   III. Godfrey,
    Martin, *1956–*   IV. Series
    615′.1   RM138

    ISBN–13:978–94–010–7076–8   e–ISBN–13:978–94–009–1295–3
    DOI:10.1007/978–94–009–1295–3

Published in the USA by
MTP Press
A division of Kluwer Academic Publishers
101 Philip Drive
Norwell, MA 02061, USA

Library of Congress Cataloging in Publication Data

Fry, John, 1922–
    Commonsense use of medicines.

    (Commonsense series)
    Includes index.
    1. Chemotherapy—Outlines, syllabi, etc. I. Trounce,
J. R. (John Reginald) II. Godfrey, Martin, MB ChB.
III. Title. IV. Series. [DNLM: 1. Drug Therapy—
handbooks. 2. Drugs—administration & dosage—hand-
books. QV 39 F946c]
RM262.F79 1987   615.5′8′0202   87-2963
ISBN–13:978–94–010–7076–8

Typeset and printed by Butler & Tanner Ltd, Frome and London

CONTENTS

PREFACE

We share with our colleagues the difficulties presented by the increasing volume of drugs available for our use in the care of patients.

The introduction of new and effective preparations has added to our problems both in keeping up to date and, paradoxically, in their proper selection and use. There are yet further difficulties in general practice because of the nature of the diseases and situations encountered; uncertainties in the preciseness of diagnosis, in the likely course and outcome of diseases and in the particular characteristics of the individual patient.

We have attempted to ease these difficulties by adopting a logical but simplistic schematic approach to the choice of medicines for 14 selected common conditions.

Our approach includes:

- statements of knowledge and understanding of the conditions;
- analyses of the most suitable available drugs;
- setting objectives and principles for management;
- suggested treatment plans.

The suggestions are, of course, our own and may not be completely acceptable to some of our readers, but in creating this schematic approach our intention has been that those who follow it will be able to select from alternative preparations with satisfactory results.

John Fry
John Trounce
Martin Godfrey

1　BASICS

Prescribing a drug is an important part of the consultation process and it has always been so. Patients seek some token or form of therapy to cure or relieve symptoms. There are ever increasing numbers of drugs to choose from, more effective and more specific in their actions than ever before, but which also carry potentially unpleasant and serious side effects; skill in prescribing becomes more and more important.

Of course, the consultation includes much more than a prescription. It provides human face-to-face and eye-to-eye contact, with the patient presenting his or her symptoms, problems and anxieties and with the physician listening, assessing, diagnosing and explaining the nature of the disorder and its management. In addition to diagnosis and treatment, the consultation should include advice on personal health promotion and disease avoidance and prevention.

However, even in these modern times with emphasis on controlled prescribing in British general practice, around two-thirds of consultations include the writing of a prescription. In addition there are many more prescriptions for 'repeat' items for continuing treatment and for 'unseen' patients seeking medication for symptoms which they do not believe merit a consultation.

EXTENT AND COSTS OF PRESCRIBING

General practice prescribing is also important because of its high cost to the National Health Service (NHS). General practice prescriptions amount to a tenth of the total cost of the NHS, now (1987) almost £2000 million a year, and hospital prescribing costs another £400 million annually. In 1987 the extent and costs of prescribing in the NHS are:

- seven prescriptions per person per year
- the cost of each prescription is approximately £4.25
- the cost of prescribing is £30 for every man, woman and child
- each general practitioner prescribes over £60 000 worth of drugs

WHY ARE PRESCRIPTIONS WRITTEN?

'To cure sometimes
To relieve often
To comfort always
To prevent hopefully'

Cures in medicine can still only be achieved 'sometimes' – by, for example, specific antibiotics.

Relief should now be possible with modern drugs for most symptoms.

Comfort must be the essence of good personal care and must be part of all consultations and contacts; it requires no drugs or potions only human kindness, concern and understanding.

Prevention, as understood by primary prevention through active immunization, is but a part of better health through self-help achieved through adherence to well-known rules of health promotion.

DIFFICULTIES

Although prescribing is such a common part of general practice it presents considerable difficulties in rationale and methodology. These relate to the very nature of general practice and the presenting problems:

- general practice is the primary level of medical care dealing with the diseases that commonly occur in the community with emphasis on minor and chronic conditions

- a precise diagnosis, substantiated by specific investigations of a disease whose causation and processes are well understood, is exceptional in general practice. Often the general practitioner has to make a diagnosis based on a rapid clinical assessment and apply treatment accordingly

- fortunately most of the common (minor) conditions of general practice are self-limiting and self-resolving but their course may at times be unpredictable, therefore drugs will not have major curative roles, but can provide relief and comfort. Many chronic conditions too are of uncertain cause and course, again specific cures cannot be expected

- paradoxically, more and better drugs create greater problems of understanding of selection and of use

It is necessary, therefore, to approach the subject logically and rationally: first, understanding the disease; second, defining objectives and principles of management; and third, becoming familiar with a selection of available drugs.

UNDERSTANDING THE DISEASE

Three questions must be asked about a disease before deciding on treatment.

what is it?

- we know enough about most diseases to make hypotheses as to their pathology and significance

who gets it and when?

- epidemiological data provide an appreciation of the prevalence and distribution of the condition

what happens?

knowledge of the natural history, the likely course and outcome of the disease, is important before commencing treatment. Benign self-limiting conditions do not need strong medicines whilst life-threatening situations demand instant effective measures. Chronic conditions require therapies appropriate to the stage and effects of the long-term disease process.

FORMULATION OF TREATMENT

objectives

- these must be appropriate for the individual patient and the disease

principles of treatment

- these must include all possible measures likely to achieve recovery and good health – among these will be many non-pharmacological steps

KNOWLEDGE OF DRUGS

Before deciding on which particular drugs to prescribe more general information is required about each group of drugs:

what are they?

- their formulation and grouping

how do they act?

- the ways in which they work and the effects that they produce

effects?

- their benefits
- their risks

which to choose?

- the type of drug
- the particular drug in a group
- a choice has to be made – what to select and why

how to use?

- having made a choice there are best ways of using the preparation

We follow this sequence for each of the common clinical conditions/situations that we have selected.

CAUTIONS

Whatever drug is used and for whatever condition there are words of caution that should be heeded.

- beware of over-enthusiastic over-expectations with the treatment
- beware of failing to pause to assess/reassess progress
- beware of over-prescribing and polypharmacy
- beware of lack of self-critical evaluation

2 ARTHRITIS

WHAT IS IT?
- an inflammation of joints
- **two main types**
  osteoarthrosis
  rheumatoid arthritis
- **other types** include juvenile arthritis, psoriatic arthritis, gout

osteoarthritis
- a degenerative condition with
  primary breakdown of cartilage
  secondary bony changes with loss of
  joint function

cause
- unknown but may be an underlying metabolic defect
- may be generalized or in one or two joints
- main joints affected
  thumb: metacarpo-phalangeal
  spine: cervical and lumbar
  knees
  hips

clinical features
- pain and stiffness worse at end of day
- a symmetrical involvement

rheumatoid arthritis
- **systemic** inflammatory disease of connective tissues
- main effects on **joints**

- chronic inflammation leading to tissue damage and necrosis with repair by fibrosis

cause
- multifactorial with strong autoimmune element
- joints affected usually symmetrically

  hands

  knees

  feet

clinical features
- joint pain and stiffness worse in morning
- other tissues affected in tendons and bursae, lungs, heart, reticuloendothelial system, kidneys and eyes

WHO GETS IT AND WHEN?
- arthritis is common

Annual prevalence of polyarthritis in a general practice population of 2500	
osteoarthrosis	60
rheumatoid arthritis	13
gout	5
psoriatic	2
other sero-negative arthritis	1
less than 1 per year	
infective and viral	1 in 3 years
anaphylactoid	1 in 5 years
collagen disease	1 in 10 years
rheumatic fever	1 in 20 years

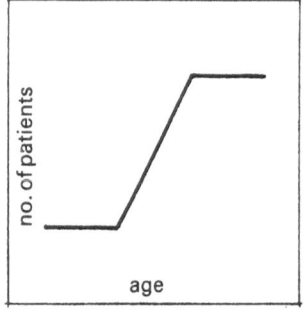

- **osteoarthritis** is a disorder associated with ageing and/or after-effects of trauma

  M = F

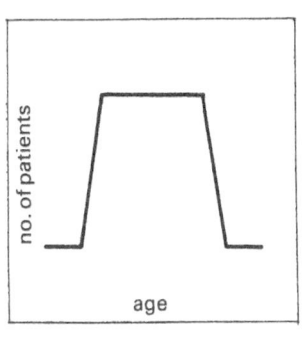

- **rheumatoid arthritis** can occur at any age but maximal incidence at 20–60

  F > M by 3:1

WHAT HAPPENS?

osteoarthritis

- often progressive with increasing symptoms and disability
- course may be episodic with flares and remissions

rheumatoid arthritis

- condition may remit at any time

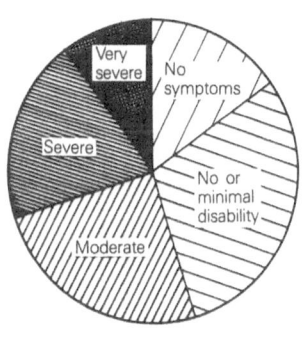

- **outcomes** may range from no disability to very severe disability

- **course** may be of various types

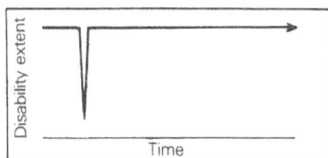

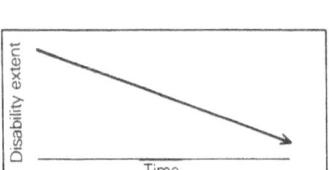

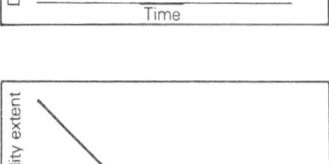

ARTHRITIS: A RECAP

- two main types
- osteoarthritis
  only joints affected with functional disability and pain
- rheumatoid arthritis
  a systemic disease
  may affect other organs as well as joints
  may be life threatening as well as disabling

WHAT TREATMENT?

objectives

- to control pain
- to prevent disability
- to control disease process, if possible
- to maintain function, encourage independence and arrange rehabilitation

DRUGS

NON-STEROIDAL ANTI-INFLAMMATORY AGENTS (NSAIA)

what are they and how do they act?
- inhibit the enzyme cyclo-oxygenase which is concerned with the synthesis of prostaglandins and thromboxane in the tissues
- relieve pain, stiffness, swelling and inflammation

effects

benefits
- **symptomatic relief** in rheumatoid and osteoarthritis, in gout and in soft tissue injuries – they do *not* alter the underlying disease process in arthritis

risks

- **gastrointestinal**

    dyspepsia

    gastric bleeding

    peptic ulcer perforation

    more common in over 60s and in women

    (do NOT use in persons with peptic ulcers)

- **bronchospasm** uncommon but can occur in asthmatics from reduced production of prostaglandin

- **fluid retention**

    can precipitate cardiac failure in at-risk subjects

    can precipitate renal failure

    (do NOT use in impaired renal function)

- **rashes**

- **CNS**

    headaches

    dizziness

    (do NOT use in last 3 months of pregnancy; ibuprofen if really necessary)

interactions

- can reverse effects of:

    diuretics

    anti-hypertensive agents

- can increase effects of:

    warfarin

    oral hypoglycaemic agents

    anticonvulsants

    (NSAIAs are generally safe if used with due attention to possible risks)

what NSAIA are available?   • large choice (only selected list given)

well established   • **aspirin**

cheap and effective

short acting (up to 4 h)

high dosage required for anti-
inflammatory effects with increased
risks of side effects
300–900 mg four hourly

(soluble aspirin pleasant to take but can
still cause gastric bleeding)

• **indomethacin**

capsules are cheap and effective
appreciable incidence of side effects

commence with small dosage 25 mg
twice daily and increase gradually to
150 mg daily

suppositories (100 mg) useful for night
pain

more recent   • **ibuprofen**

short action

dose-related side effects

less effective at lower dosage

200–400 mg three or four times per day

• **diclofenac**

25–50 mg eight hourly

• **naproxen**

250–500 mg 12 hourly

• **piroxicam**

10–20 mg once daily

pro-drug   • **fenbufen**

600 mg at night with 300 mg more if
necessary

- **benorylate** (aspirin/paracetamol ester) 1.5–2 g eight hourly

  (these are broken down in gut wall and liver releasing active components and avoiding gastric irritation)

which to use?

- no 'best buy'
- choice is personal and rests on experience, cost, dosage-frequency and risks of side effects

- variable patient-responses

how to use?

practical points

- start with standard dosage in young and middle aged but low dose in elderly

- if no response after 3 weeks do not go above recommended dose but switch to another NSAIA or other treatment

- take with or after food
- only use one NSAIA at a time
- for **morning stiffness** use long-acting preparation or a suppository at night, or rapidly acting drug on waking (aspirin or ibuprofen)

- use with special care in elderly as risks from fluid retention and gastric bleeding

- do NOT use as non-specific anodyne

- if indicated in patients with history of dyspepsia use ibuprofen, fenbufen or benorylate or combine with antacid or H_2 antagonist

- do NOT use with renal or liver disease

simple analgesics (use with NSAIAs for pain control)

- paracetamol 1 g every 4–6 hours

- co-proxamol (paracetamol 325 mg and dextropropoxyphene 32.5 mg per tablet) is controversial (dangerous in overdosage)

DRUGS THAT ALTER THE RHEUMATOID PROCESS

what are they and how do they work?

- heterogenous group of drugs which suppress the rheumatoid process in ways not fully understood
- **penicillamine** dissociates macroglobulins
- **gold** inhibits the immune process
- **chloroquine** stabilizes lysosomes

effects

benefits

- improvements in rheumatoid arthritis within 3 months in:

  75% on gold or penicillamine

  50% on chloroquine

risks

- all have possible side-effects and require careful monitoring. Don't start in pregnancy
- **penicillamine** side-effects common, one third stop treatment

  thrombocytopoenia in 25% therefore do full blood count every 2 weeks for 3 months and then monthly. If platelets <100 000 stop drug, and if recovery, then start at half dose but stop if platelets fall

  leucopoenia: stop treatment, and if recovery restart at half dose with care

  proteinuria: test weekly – if heavy stop and do not restart; if mild stop and if recovery then half dose

  rashes: if early in treatment, stop and restart when clear;

  if late in treatment, stop and do not restart
  loss of taste: recovers, do not stop drug

  (do NOT use in renal or liver disease)

- **gold** adverse effects common, one third stop treatment

  rashes: stop and do not restart

proteinuria: test on each visit
stop and resume when clear with low
dose (20 mg). If persistent, abandon
treatment

thrombocytopoenia or leucopoenia:
check blood before each treatment and
if present, stop treatment

stomatitis recovers on stopping drug

arthritis may be exacerbated
(do NOT use in renal disease, SLE or
pregnancy)

- **chloroquine**

  retinal damage, usually after 1 year of
  treatment: get ophthalmological
  opinion before starting and every 6
  months

(do NOT use in elderly)

what to use?

- no single preferred drug
- **chloroquine** is least effective so use in less
  severe rheumatoid arthritis
- **penicillamine and gold** equally effective
  but gold is given by injection
- *note:* ALL must be carefully monitored

how to use?

- Only effective in **active** rheumatoid
  arthritis
- **chloroquine** also in SLE and discoid lupus
- **penicillamine** by mouth and before food

  initial dose 125 mg daily for 1 month

  increase by 125 mg daily every 6 weeks
  to maximum of 750 mg daily with
  expected response in 2–3 months

- **sodium aurothiomalate** by deep i.m. injection weekly

    start with 10 mg weekly, then 20 mg weekly, then 50 mg weekly until remission or total of 1 g given

    thereafter 50 mg monthly for maintenance

    response should be noted within 3 months

    (gold is becoming less popular because of appreciable side effects and need for injection)

- **chloroquine sulphate** 200 mg after food once daily

OTHER DRUGS

azathioprine

- cytotoxic immunosuppressive – may act as gold and penicillamine
- dose: 2.0 mg/kg body weight/day daily by mouth
- myelotoxic: check blood weekly for first 8 weeks and then monthly

sulphasalazine

- may achieve relief in resistant rheumatoid arthritis
- dose: initial 0.5 g daily increasing by 0.5 g per week to 2 g daily

corticosteroids: systemic (by mouth)

benefits

- rapid relief of symptoms in rheumatoid arthritis

risks

- long-term use disappointing because increasing dosage may be required with high incidence of adverse effects

	• disease process is not arrested and appreciable risk of side effects and complications with long use
how to use?	• only in progressive disease and where unresponsive to other treatments
	• lowest effective dose of prednisolone (<10 mg daily)
	• reduce gradually to avoid relapse

córticosteroids: local (e.g. by intra-articular injection)

how to use?	• suitable for
	soft tissue lesions (tennis elbow, capsulitis, tendinitis)
	single painful rheumatoid or osteo-arthritic joints
	• can use:
	hydrocortisone acetate (short duration)
	methyl prednisolone acetate (long duration)
risks	• results are unpredictable
	• need for strict aseptic precautions
	• possible increase in rate of joint deterioration

osteoarthritis

general measures

- important, as weight reduction for weight-bearing joints (knees and hips), supports for neck and back, physiotherapy
- there are no specific treatments and aims are pain relief and reduction of inflammation

pain relief = analgesics

- *aspirin* also has some anti-inflammatory actions 300–900 mg four to six hourly and up to 3–4 g daily
- *paracetamol* if dyspepsia troublesome
    1 g six hourly
- *co-proxamol* of questionable use because of danger of overdose and possible dependence

    two tablets six hourly as required

control of joint inflammatory reactions

- *NSAIA:*
  indomethacin commence with 25 mg twice daily and go up to 150 mg daily if necessary

    If no response within 3–4 weeks, then other NSAIAs can be tried (see p. 10)
- *intra-articular steroid injections* may relieve pain dramatically in short term
  repeated injections may lead to damage to cartilage and bone
- surgery often achieves complete 'cure' by *joint replacement* most successful for arthritis of hip

rheumatoid arthritis

- *note* that arthritis is part of the rheumatoid process, with various grades and outcomes

general measures

- include maintenance of health, appropriate rest and exercises, splintage and appliances

mild and moderate cases

- as for osteoarthritis

  aspirin

  NSAIAs

- analgesics like paracetamol or co-proxamol may be helpful during painful periods

progressive

- control of rheumatoid process

  oral penicillamine – start with 125 mg daily and increase slowly to maximum 750 mg

  intramuscular gold (sodium aurothiomalate) 10 mg rising to 50 mg weekly or monthly
  (regular injections and careful monitoring)

- *note:* beneficial response may be slow and not be fully apparent for 3 months
- *note:* both drugs have possible serious side effects, as blood disorders and renal damage (blood and urine must be monitored)

severe

- consider systemic (oral) steroids but though relief may be dramatic, dangerous long-term side-effects are likely and it is difficult to withdraw the drug once started
- local intra-articular injections of steroids may relieve acute exacerbations
- consider immunosuppressive drugs or sulphasalazine in difficult cases
- surgery may be helpful to remove inflamed tissues, to replace or to fix joints

3   DUODENAL ULCER

WHAT IS IT?

- a **clinical syndrome**
- **diagnosis** must be confirmed by barium meal and/or endoscopy

causes

- a **'diathesis'**: some individuals are prone to duodenal ulceration with a family history, in blood group O and are non-secretors (no blood group activity in intestinal secretions)
- production of excess gastric acid and pepsin
- defective duodenal mucosal defence mechanisms that prevent autodigestion by acid and pepsin
- trigger factors such as irritants – smoking, alcohol, steroids and NSAIAs

WHO GETS IT WHEN?

age prevalence

- condition of early adult life 25–35
- M > F by 3:1
- affects 10% of adults

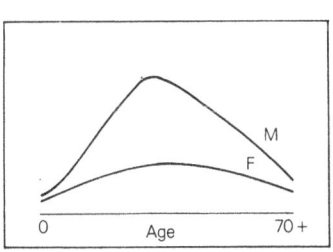

DU: general practice with 2500 patients

• new cases	5–10
• patients consulting	35
• patients with history of DU	106

• **annual prevalence** in a general practice of 2500

WHAT HAPPENS?

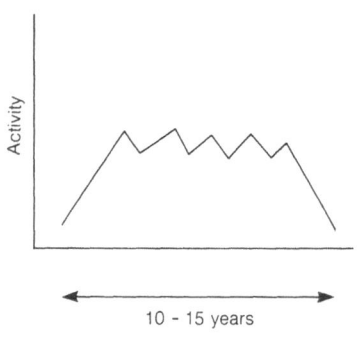

Activity

10 - 15 years

• a condition of **remissions and recurrences**
• tendency for **eventual 'spontaneous cure'** 75% will eventually remain healed after 10–15 years and not recur

with or without treatment

• 40% heal in 4 weeks
• 80% heal in 8 weeks
• 75% recur in 1 year

attacks

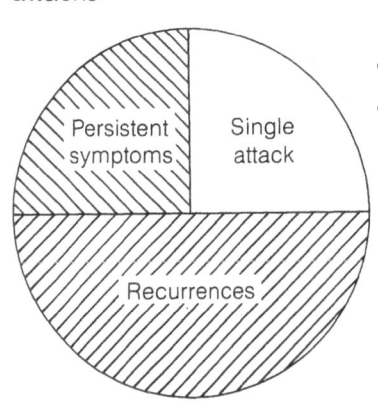

Persistent symptoms | Single attack

Recurrences

• 25% suffer single attack with no recurrence
• 50% suffer recurrent episodic attacks
• 25% suffer persistent symptoms

complications
- bleeding in 17%
- perforation in 3%
- pyloric stenosis in <1%

DUODENAL ULCER: RECAP

- condition affecting prone individuals
- precise cause unknown but related to gastric hyperacidity and defective mucosal barrier
- likely natural history is for recurrent attacks over 10–15 years that will eventually cease spontaneously

---

WHAT TREATMENT?

---

objectives
- to relieve symptoms
- to promote healing
- to prevent recurrences
- to prevent complications

DRUGS
ANTACIDS

what are they and how do they act?
- antacids buffer and neutralize gastric hydrochloric acid
- by raising intragastric pH they reduce irritation of the ulcer and inactivate some peptic enzymes – this effect on gastric acidity is relatively transient

effects

benefits
- rapid relief of symptoms in duodenal ulcer
- healing only with large and frequent doses

adverse effects
- diarrhoea with magnesium salts

| | • distension and belching with sodium bicarbonate |
| | • constipation with aluminium hydroxide |

risks

- low risk potential generally
- do NOT use **sodium-containing antacids** in heart failure, renal failure and late pregnancy because of dangers of sodium overload
- **calcium salts** rarely cause hypercalcaemia in high dosage
- **magnesium and aluminium retention** can occur in renal failure

interactions

- antacids may interfere with absorption of other drugs (as digoxin, indomethacin, isoniazid, tetracycline) if taken at same time
- antacids may also cause enteric coated tablets to dissolve prematurely in the stomach

what is available?

- magnesium trisilicate mixture (also contains sodium bicarbonate and tablets may further contain aluminium hydroxide)
- aluminium hydroxide (tablets or mixture)
- **all are cheap and generally effective**

There are many other preparations available. The following may be useful for special purposes:
- **Maalox Concentrate** tablets or suspension
  (magnesium trisilicate and aluminium hydroxide)
  use when sodium free suspension indicated, *or*
  when magnesium and aluminium salts required in combination

- **Gaviscon** tablets or suspension

- **Gastrocote** tablets

  both contain alginic acid, magnesium trisilicate, aluminium hydroxide and sodium bicarbonate

  form foam layer on gastric or oesophageal mucosa

  indicated in peptic oesophagitis

- **Mucaine**

  (suspension of aluminium and magnesium hydroxides and oxethazaine)

  useful in peptic oesophagitis because of the local anaesthetic effects of oxethazaine

  taken before a meal

which to use?
- selection of antacid is not critical
- magnesium trisilicate and aluminium hydroxide preparations are cheap, effective and have minimal side-effects
- chewed tablets have more prolonged effect than liquid preparations

how to use?
- **symptom control:** one or two tablets or 10–15 ml of magnesium trisilicate or aluminium hydroxide after meal and at bedtime
- **promotion of healing:** large dose 30 ml/two to four tablets of magnesium trisilicate or aluminium hydroxide mixture/tablets, 1 and 3 h after meals and at bedtime

  further doses in night if awakened
- **in peptic oesophagitis:** Gaviscon after meals and at bedtime; Mucaine before meals and at bedtime

H_2 RECEPTOR ANTAGONISTS

what are they and how do they act?
- histamine stimulates gastric parietal cells to release hydrochloric acid – this is the final step in a process involving acetylcholine release by vagus nerves and gastrin

- H$_2$ antagonists act by blocking this final
  step and reduce acid secretion by 80%

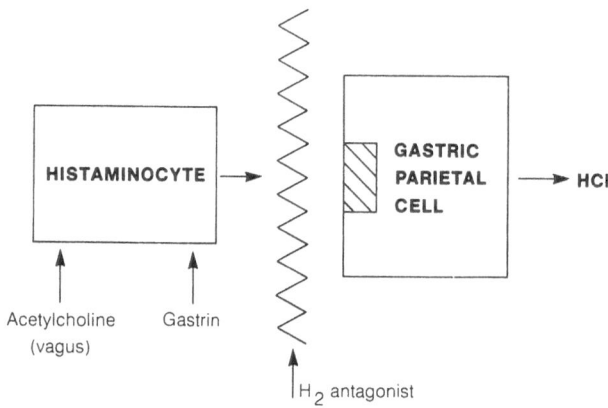

what is available?

- cimetidine
- ranitidine
- famotidine

effects
benefits

- rapid relief of symptoms followed by ulcer
  healing in 70–80%
- relapse likely if drugs withdrawn before
  complete healing
- also beneficial in
  peptic oesophagitis
  stress ulcers
  Zollinger–Ellison syndrome
  (do NOT use for vague non-ulcer
  dyspepsias)

risks

- low risk rates and few side-effects
- limited experience shows famotidine is
  very similar to ranitidine

cimetidine	ranitidine
Rare binding to androgen receptors	
• gynaecomastia	
• impotence	
Inhibits breakdown of other drugs	No evidence of such effects
• warfarin	
• phenytoin	
• aminophylline	
Rare confusion in elderly	
Low dose in renal impairment	Low dose in renal impairment

which to use?
- little to choose between them
- ranitidine in young men

how to use?
- cimetidine 400 mg twice daily after meals or 800 mg at night
- ranitidine 150 mg twice daily after meals or 300 mg at night
- symptoms should disappear rapidly if diagnosis correct
- continue at above dosage for 6 weeks to ensure healing
- thereafter for a further 3 months
  cimetidine 400 mg at night
  ranitidine 150 mg at night
- famotidine use is similar to ranitidine with twice daily dosage

with relapse
- 70% are likely to relapse in 12 months once treatment stops
- if episodic: treat symptoms as they arise
- if frequent and prolonged: long-term treatment with single night dose

- if gastric ulcer also present: endoscope at end of course of treatment to ensure healing and exclude gastric cancer, whose symptoms may be relieved temporarily

ANTI-CHOLINERGICS

what are they and how do they act?

- competitively inhibit muscarinic cholinergic receptors and reduce vagal stimulated acid secretion
- volume rather than pH of gastric acid secretion is diminished
- gastric motility reduced and emptying time prolonged
- non-selective anti-cholinergic actions cause troublesome side-effects
- new product, pirenzepine, is a selective anti-cholinergic with few side-effects

effects

benefits

- older anticholinergics produced some symptomatic relief but had no effect on ulcer healing
- pirenzepine healing effects are as good as H_2 antagonists

Risks and side effects

- due to cholinergic blockade
   dry mouth
   difficulties with accommodation (note: glaucoma risk)
   constipation
   urinary retention (especially in older men)
(insignificant with pirenzepine)

how to use?

- start with pirenzepine 50 mg twice daily and increase if necessary to three times daily

- can be combined with antacids and delay in gastric emptying will prolong their effects
- usual period of use is 6 weeks, maximum should be 3 months

SITE PROTECTIVE AGENTS

what are they and how do they act?
- coat the ulcer base and protect it from acid and pepsin

> - bismuth chelate (De-Nol) is a colloidal bismuth compound
> - sucralfate (Antepsin) is a complex of sulphated sucrose and aluminium hydroxide

effects

benefits
- relieve symptoms and promote ulcer healing
- as effective as H_2 antagonists

risks and adverse effects
- bismuth chelate liquid has unpleasant taste, tablets are available
  stools and tongue blackened
  constipation
  do NOT use in renal failure
  do NOT use with milk or antacids as they neutralize action

how to use?
- bismuth chelate (120 mg (5 ml) in 15 ml water) four times a day $\frac{1}{2}$ h before three main meals and 2 h after the last for 1 month (unpleasant taste: one 120 mg tablet may be preferred, crushed in mouth and washed down with water)
- sucralfate 1 g four times a day 1 h before three meals and at bedtime for 6–12 weeks (can increase to 2 g dose)

SURGERY

indications

- failed medical treatment
- complications
  bleeding
  perforation
  stenosis
- possible gastric cancer

operations

- **vagotomy** (duodenal ulcer)
  section of vagal nerves to reduce gastric
    and pepsin production
  truncal and drainage or
  selective and no drainage
- **gastrectomy** (gastric and some duodenal
  ulcers)

results

recurrence

- 5–15% after vagotomy
- <5% after gastrectomy

mortality

- <1% after vagotomy
- 1–3% after gastrectomy

complications

- after gastrectomy
  anaemia
  weight loss
  malabsorption and deficiencies

TREATMENT PLAN

general measures
- advice that is probably helpful
  stop smoking
  take small frequent meals
  avoid known aggravating foods as alcohol, coffee, tea, spices, curries

- important to explain nature and likely course of intermittent attacks and ultimate natural resolution

- important to explain the treatment regime to be used and actions and purposes of the drugs

- do not use specific drugs until diagnosis confirmed by radiology and/or endoscopy

mild episodic attacks
- alkalis
  chew two tablets after meals or when pain present and at bedtime of:
  aluminium hydroxide, *or*
  magnesium trisilicate, *or*
  mixtures of these and other alkalis

persistent or recurring (frequently)
- a stage plan is useful

- *1st line: H₂ receptor antagonists*
  for 6–8 weeks and then single bedtime dose for 3 months of:
  cimetidine 400 mg twice daily, *or*
  ranitidine 150 mg twice daily, *or*
  famotidine
  note: 70% relapse in a year: decision then to be made whether to treat *ad hoc* or to use small dosage long term)

- *2nd line: site protectives* (for frequent relapsers)
  bismuth chelate 120 mg before meals and at night for 1 month, *or*
  sucralfate 1 g before meals and at night for 6–12 weeks

- *3rd line: anticholinergic*
  pirenzepine 50 mg twice daily before meals for 6–12 weeks

'medical failures'
- a few will continue to suffer continuing symptoms, or complications, in spite of long-term medication

- *surgery* must then be considered and it is wrong to delay overlong

4

DIARRHOEA: ACUTE AND CHRONIC

WHAT IS IT?

- **Diarrhoea** is a broad term for a common clinical presentation with
    frequent bowel actions
    fluid-soft stools

- **two types**
    most are **acute** and self-limiting
    a few are **chronic** with major
        management problems

diagnosis

- usually on clinical assessment

- investigations
    rarely helpful in **acute** diarrhoea
    must be undertaken in all **chronic**
        diarrhoea

- feces examination for
    specific pathogens
    occult blood
    fat + in malabsorption

- endoscopy
    sigmoidoscopy and/or colonoscopy for
        possible inflammatory or neoplastic
        lesions

- radiology
    barium enema in all chronic diarrhoeas

causes

acute

- mostly of uncertain cause

- some **infective**
    - ? bacteria: *E. coli*
    - salmonella
    - shigella
    - *Campylobacter*
    - ? protozoal: amoebiasis
    - *Giardia lamblia*

- **toxaemic**

- **remote conditions**
    - upper respiratory infections in children
    - acute appendicitis

- **fecal impaction**

chronic

- **inflammatory**
    - ulcerative colitis
    - Crohn's disease

- **cancer of large bowel**

- **irritable bowel syndrome** (IBS)

- **diverticular disease**

- **drug effects**
    - laxatives
    - antibiotics

WHO GETS IT AND WHEN?

- different types likely to occur at different ages

young

- acute gastroenteritis
- coeliac disease
- fibrocystic disease
- intussusception
- laxative misuse
- 'normal'

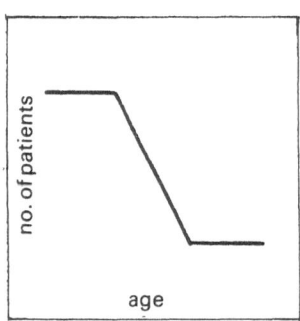

no. of patients

age

mid age

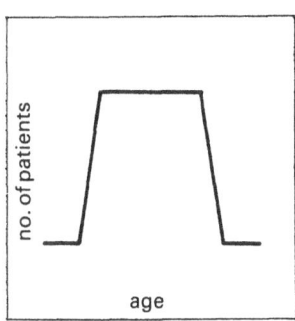

- IBS
- ulcerative colitis
- Crohn's disease
- malabsorption syndromes
- drug induced
- cancer

old

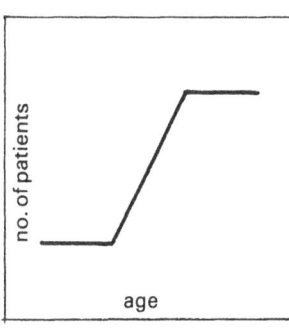

- cancer
- diverticular disease
- fecal impaction
- drug induced
- **annual prevalence** in a general practice of 2500

Annual prevalence of conditions presenting as 'diarrhoea' in a general practice of 2500 persons

Acute intestinal infections	125
'Irritable bowel syndrome'	50
Iatrogenic drug reactions	10
Diverticular disease	10
Fecal impaction	4
Colitis	3
Cancer	1
Fibrocystic disease	1
Less than 1 per year	
Acute abdomen	2 in 3 years
Coeliac disease and other malabsorption disorders	1 in 2 years
Crohn's disease	1 in 5 years
Ischaemic bowel disease	1 in 7 years

WHAT HAPPENS?

acute diarrhoea

- most are self-limiting and clear naturally in 2 or 3 days
- if not then an unusual specific cause should be considered

- dangers are:
   fluid-electrolyte depletion
   toxicity from infection

chronic diarrhoea

- course depends on cause and type
- some may continue for years with specific complications

DIARRHOEA: RECAP

- a common condition
- significance depends on the causes
- in most **acute diarrhoeas** no specific cause is found even with investigations, but fortunately most resolve in a few days
- dangers are in loss of fluid and electrolytes, especially if accompanied by vomiting
- **chronic diarrhoea** is a clinical challenge that may require detailed investigation

---

WHAT TREATMENT?

---

objectives
acute

- to manage the attack
- to prevent complications
- to determine cause and source if appropriate
- prevent spread, if appropriate

chronic

- to discover cause and nature of condition
- to apply specific treatment

DRUGS IN ACUTE DIARRHOEA

FLUIDS AND ELECTROLYTES

what and why?

- fluid and electrolyte balance must be maintained in **acute** diarrhoea until recovery occurs

diet

- clear fluids only for 24–48 h

- in **mild** cases glucose and water mixtures or Lucozade are appropriate

- in infants, young children and elderly **severe** depletion of fluids and electrolytes can occur and especially prepared mixtures of glucose and electrolytes may be indicated

what available?

> - **sodium chloride and glucose oral powder compound BNF**
> - **Dioralyte sachets** (sodium chloride, potassium chloride, sodium bicarbonate and glucose)
> - **Rehidrat sachets** (sodium chloride, potassium chloride, sodium bicarbonate, glucose, sucrose and fructose)

how to use?

- **Dioralyte**: one sachet dissolved in 200 ml freshly boiled water
  infants: 150 ml/kg daily
  children and adults: 40 ml/kg daily

- **Rehidrat**: one sachet dissolved in 250 ml water 150 ml/kg daily

- **after 24 h in infants**
  reintroduce $\frac{1}{4}$ strength milk diluted with boiled water and build up to full strength over 3 days (relapse at this stage suggests temporary milk sensitivity)

ANTIBIOTICS

Only indicated in **acute** diarrhoea for specific infections or where evidence of systemic infection as in typhoid

DRUGS IN CHRONIC DIARRHOEA/INFLAMMATORY BOWEL DISEASE

STEROIDS IN ULCERATIVE COLITIS

what are they and how do they act?
- non-specific anti-inflammatory actions in ulcerative colitis and Crohn's disease
- help to bring attack under control

effects

benefits
- symptoms controlled in most patients within 2–3 weeks

risks
- as for all steroids

what available?

> - prednisolone tablets
> - prednisolone retention enemas (some absorbed from bowel)
> - prednisolone suppositories
> - Colifoam (hydrocortisone foam)

which to use and how?
- if condition predominantly affects the **rectum** (blood and mucus in stools but insignificant diarrhoea) then prednisolone **enemas** (or suppositories or Colifoam) at night and retained for at least an hour – for up to 1 month or until remission occurs. **Suppositories** effective only with minimal disease
- if disease is more extensive affecting **colon** (liquid stools) prednisolone tablets 40 mg daily and gradually reducing over 1 month

SULPHASALAZINE IN ULCERATIVE COLITIS

what is it and how does it act?
- a combination of sulphapyridine and 5-aminosalicylic acid
- is split in the gut when the 5-aminosalicylic acid exerts an anti-inflammatory effect

effects

benefits
- produces remissions in mild attacks
- maintains remission

risks
- nausea – dose related
- sulphapyridine acetylated and more than half population are slow acetylators with possible increased incidence of **side-effects** such as nausea, headache, vomiting, vertigo
- **hypersensitivity** – blood dyscrasias
- reversible lowered sperm counts during treatment
- do NOT use in persons with known sulpha or salicylate sensitivities; glucose-6-phosphate dehydrogenase deficiency; and in liver and renal diseases

what to use?
- **sulphasalazine** unless known 'sulpha' intolerance when **mesalazine**, which only contains 5-aminosalicylic acid, can be used

how to use?
- **sulphasalazine**
  1·0 g orally every 6 h until remission
  1·0 g twice daily for maintenance
  (effective in 75%)
- **mesalazine** (controlled release tablets)
  1·2 to 2·4 g in divided doses daily and swallowed whole

- **full blood counts** at start and monthly for first 3 months (to pick up blood dyscrasias)

what happens?

course

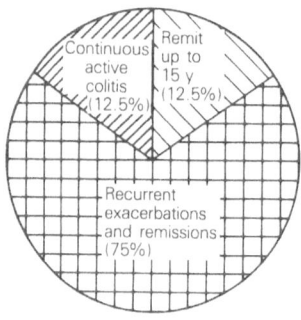

- 75% recurrent remissions and exacerbations
- 12·5% continuous colitis
- 12·5% remit for 15 years +

complications

- 20% cancer after 20 years (transverse and ascending colon)
- 25% polyarthritis
- reduced life expectation

DRUGS USED IN CROHN'S DISEASE

management

- similar to ulcerative colitis but less satisfactory, Crohn's disease is difficult to treat

systemic steroids

- only for acute attacks (especially small bowel)
- not long term

sulphasalazine

- may help in colonic involvement
- best for mild-moderate attacks
- does not prevent relapses

azathioprine	• cytotoxic drug
	• for resistant cases, allows reduction of steroid dose
	• risks of bone marrow damage
	• monthly blood checks
cholestyramine	• with aluminium hydroxide and low fat diet if diarrhoea considered to be results of failure to absorb bile salts
metronidazole	• useful in perianal involvement and sometimes in colonic disease

BULKING AGENTS

bran	• 30% fibre
	• reduces intraluminal pressure and promotes propulsion of bowel contents
	• one to three tablespoonfuls mixed with food daily, and with plentiful fluid
other bulking agents	• methyl cellulose
	• ispaghula husk
	• sterculia

FLUID ADSORBENTS

| **what are they and how do they act?** | • **kaolin** and **chalk** adsorb fluid and render intestinal contents less fluid |
| | • **ispaghula husk**, **methyl cellulose** and **sterculia** also adsorb, but slowly and not helpful in acute diarrhoea |

effects

- although use is traditional no reliable evidence of any real benefit
- risks of promoting unnecessary placebo-medication
- may delay and/or mask diagnosis of serious disease in infants and children

MOTILITY INHIBITORS

what are they and how do they act?

- **opium** and **morphine** and related **codeine phosphate** and **loperamide** reduce bowel motility and allow more absorption of water
- **mebeverine** acts directly on the bowel and relaxes spasm
- **propantheline** is an anti-cholinergic and relaxes spasm

effects

benefits

- codeine and loperamide are useful in relieving diarrhoea
- mebeverine and propantheline relieve symptoms in IBS

risks

- codeine may exacerbate diverticular disease and IBS
- codeine may cause central depression in children
- codeine and loperamide must be avoided in liver disease
- they may cause bowel distension in acute ulcerative colitis
- codeine may cause constipation and dependence
- propantheline may cause anti-cholinergic effects and lead to urinary retention and glaucoma

which to use?

- codeine in adults to relieve diarrhoea (do NOT use for children)
- mebeverine to supplement bran in IBS

how to use?

- codeine phosphate: 15–60 mg four to six times daily
- loperamide in **acute** diarrhoea
    4 mg to start followed by 2 mg after each stool, to a maximum of 16 mg per day
- loperamide in **chronic** diarrhoea
    2 mg up to four times a day
- mebeverine: 135 mg three times daily before meals
- propantheline: 15 mg three times daily before meals and 30 mg at night when necessary

TREATMENT PLAN

acute diarrhoea

note:

- most acute diarrhoeas are of undetermined cause and resolve in 2 or 3 days
- try and discover any source and take public health measures
- severely dehydrated persons, particularly infants and children, and when vomiting is associated with diarrhoea making oral treatment difficult, need urgent admission to hospital for intravenous feeding
- elderly patients may be on diuretics – these should be stopped

general measures

- priority is to deal with effects of loss of fluid and electrolytes
- clear fluids only until diarrhoea ceases
- supplemental electrolyte-glucose preparations in more severe attacks
- hospital admission may be necessary in infants

drugs
- usually not required
- for control of symptoms in adults
  codeine phosphate 15–30 mg six hourly for 1 or 2 days
  loperamide 2 mg after each stool
  kaolin or chalk mixtures
- for specific infections
  (antibiotics only if specific pathogens isolated)
  giardiasis: metronidazole
                     2.0 g daily for 3 days
  Campylobacter: erythromycin
                     2 g daily for 1 week
  typhoid: chloramphenicol
                     500 mg six hourly for 2 weeks
  dysentery: antibiotics not necessary

chronic diarrhoea

note: determine diagnosis before treating

ulcerative colitis (may occur in acute, intermittent or persistent forms)

mild   (less than six stools per day and general condition
                      good)

- *steroids*
    local enemas: prednisolone (Predsol) or Colifoam when
    disease confined to rectum
    systemic: prednisolone 40 mg on first few days (when colon
                      involved) and reduce and withdraw over a month

- *sulphasalazine*
    2–4 g daily in divided doses until remission
    then 1 g twice daily for maintenance

- *mesalazine*
    1·2–2·4 g daily in divided doses
    for long term to prevent relapse

severe   (more than six stools daily and poor general
                      condition)

- ADMISSION NECESSARY

persistent

- steroids

- sulphasalazine

- mesalazine

- all drugs long term in lowest effective doses

note

- surgery may be required in severely ill or in chronic cases

- in 75% course is intermittent over years

- in 12·5% no symptoms after 5–15 years

- in 12·5% chronic persistent state

- in 20% cancer in transverse or ascending colon after 20 years

- in 25% polyarthritis

- reduced life expectancy

Crohn's disease
a systemic disease with main effects on small and large bowel,
with unpredictable course

general measures

- advise high fibre diet

drugs

- steroids (as for ulcerative colitis)
- sulphasalazine (as for ulcerative colitis)
- azathioprine may be considered in severe chronic cases

diverticular disease

bulking agents

- bran
- ispaghula
- sterculia

irritable bowel syndrome

bulking agents

drugs

- loperamide 6–8 mg daily
- mebeverine 135 mg three times daily
- all drugs in divided doses

5 CONSTIPATION

WHAT IS IT?

'Constipation' is defined as 'infrequent passage of hard feces'

- wide range of 'normal' in frequency of defecation from once per week to many times daily
- can be separated into two types **acute** and **chronic**

causes

acute

- intestinal obstruction
- painful defecation

chronic

- low bulk of food or fluid intake
- dyschezia – ignoring call to defecation
- motility (and obstructive) disorders
  irritable bowel syndrome
  ageing bowel
  diverticulosis
  long-term laxatives
- drugs – iron, aluminium, codeine, opiates, anticholinergics
- others – hypothyroid, CNS disorders

WHO GETS IT WHEN?

- a frequent symptom, everyone 'suffers' from constipation sometimes
- although very prevalent not a frequent reason for consultation in general practice (most will self-medicate)

Grades of severity

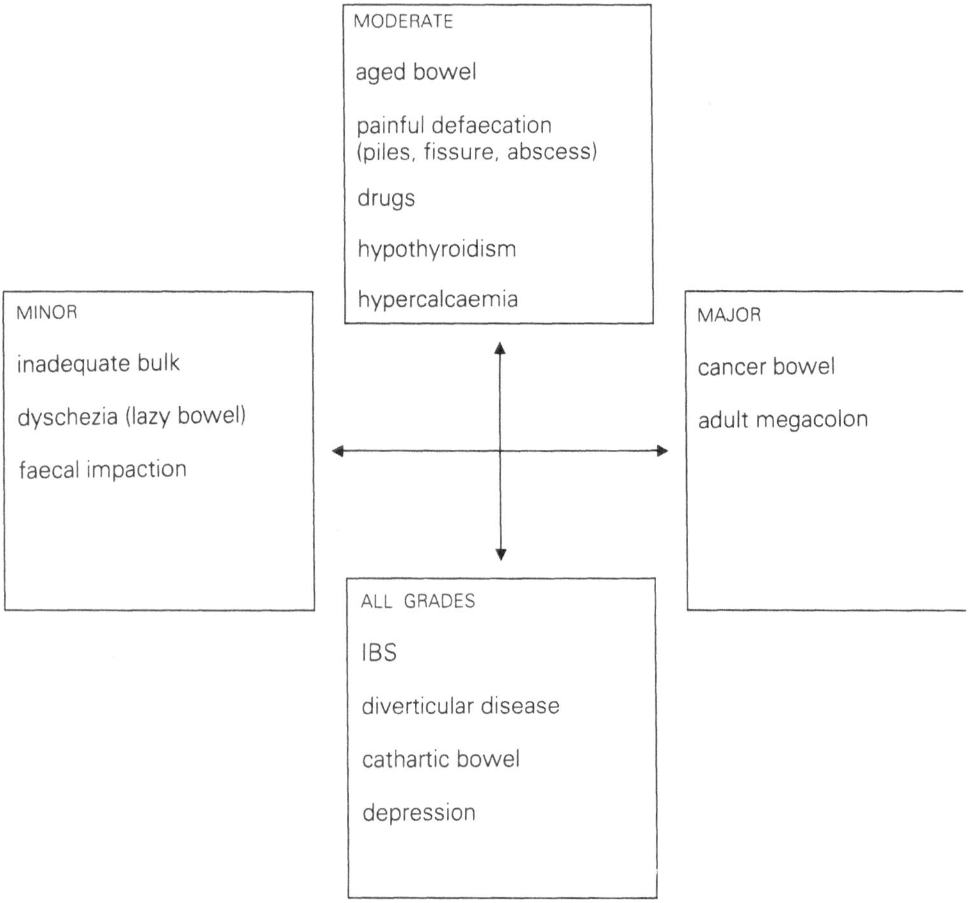

MODERATE
aged bowel
painful defaecation (piles, fissure, abscess)
drugs
hypothyroidism
hypercalcaemia
MINOR
inadequate bulk
dyschezia (lazy bowel)
faecal impaction
MAJOR
cancer bowel
adult megacolon
ALL GRADES
IBS
diverticular disease
cathartic bowel
depression

age incidence

no. of patients
age

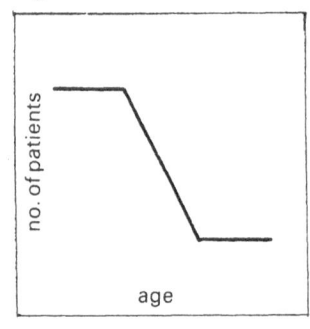

- bad habits
- painful defecation
- imaginary (parental)

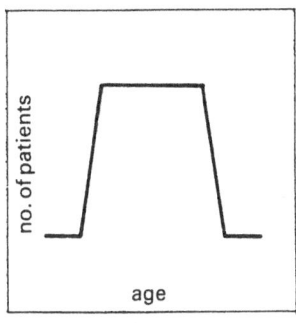

- inadequate bulk
- dyschezia (lazy bowel)
- IBS
- depression
- hypothyroidism
- piles, fissure
- cathartic bowel

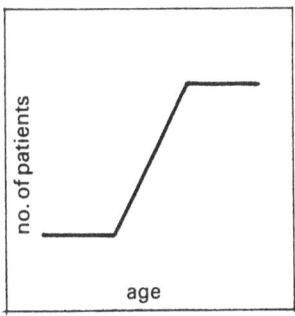

- fecal impaction
- carcinomata of large bowel
- diverticular disease

WHAT HAPPENS?

- course and outcome depend on nature and causes
- in common functional constipation, constant distension of the rectum leads to failure of stretch receptors to respond with build-up of retained hard feces

---

CONSTIPATION : A RECAP

- a frequent symptom
- many possible causes
- differentiate possible remediable 'organic' causes from 'functional' ones
- recognize iatrogenic causes

WHAT TREATMENT?

objectives
- to make a definitive diagnosis
- to pick out remediable types
- to emphasize role of self-help
- to relieve symptoms
- to restore regular painless defecation

DRUGS

BULKING AGENTS

what are they and how do they work?

plant fibre
- undigestible portion of plant that takes up water and swells within the gut – this greatly distends and stretches the bowel wall and induces useful peristalsis

bran contains	30% fibre
wholemeal bread contains	
	2.5% fibre
white bread contains	0.2% fibre

ispaghula
- prepared from seed husks and similar actions to bran

methylcellulose
- similar actions to bran

effects

benefits
- long term use in preventing constipation

48

	• lowers bowel intraluminal pressure and relieves symptoms in diverticular disease and in the irritable bowel syndrome (with constipation)
risks	• **bran** can cause unpleasant distension and wind so start with small doses
	• **ispaghula** can produce impaction of granules, if insufficient fluid is taken
which to use?	• bran is cheap and readily available (not on NHS prescription)
	• elderly patients may find ispaghula or methylcellulose more acceptable

how to give?

bran	• start with half tablespoonful daily with plenty of fluid and increase slowly to two tablespoonfuls daily.
ispaghula	• granules (Isogel): two teaspoonfuls after meals with water once or twice daily
	• sachets (Regulan): one sachet with water one to three times daily after meals
methylcellulose '450'	• three to six tablets twice daily after meals with water

note: plentiful fluid intake with all these preparations

OSMOTIC LAXATIVES: LACTULOSE

what is it and how does it work?	• a disaccharide that is broken down in the gut to release substances which retain fluid in the bowel with gas

effects

benefits
- relieves constipation
- particularly useful in children as does not cause diarrhoea
- main use in hepatic encephalopathy as it inhibits ammonia-producing organisms in the gut

risks
- do NOT use in persons with lactose intolerance

how to give?
- children < 1 year: 2.5 ml twice daily
- children 1–5 years: 5 ml twice daily
- adults: 15 ml twice daily
- in hepatic encephalopathy: 30–50 ml three times daily
- reduce as required

STOOL SOFTENERS: DOCUSATE SODIUM

what are they and how do they act?
- surface active agents which soften stool by allowing more water to penetrate

effects

benefits
- useful in initial treatment of chronic constipation (acts in about 2 days)
- useful to ease defecation in painful piles and anal fissure

risks
- may alter permeability of gut
- avoid long-term use

how to give?
- **docusate:** start with 100 mg four times daily and reduce

STIMULANT LAXATIVES

what are they and how do • increase activity of large bowel
they act?

effects

benefits • bowel action within 10 h

risks • can produce colic

• do NOT use in pregnancy and in children

• prolonged use can cause atonic bowel
and electrolyte deficiencies
(hypokalaemia)

what is available and • for short term use only
how to give? **senna** (as Senokot): adult – one tablet
at night increasing to two to four if
necessary
child (2–6 years) 2.5–5 ml elixir at
night
child (over 6 years) 5–10 ml elixir at night
bisacodyl: tablet 5–10 mg at night (avoid
taking it with milk or antacid)
suppository 10 mg on rising

SUPPOSITORIES

what are they and how do • soften feces and stimulate rectal wall and
they work? lead to emptying of rectum and colon

• rapid action

which and how to use? • many combinations

• **glycerol suppository** is usually effective

• moisten well before insertion
(**note:** different sizes for adults and children)

TREATMENT PLAN

note: first exclude any remediable cause such as neoplasm or
fecal impaction

general advice

- diet with bulk and fibre+

- habits – regular

- avoidance of long-term laxative abuse

for immediate relief

- suppositories
    glycerol
    bisacodyl

- enema

for occasional use

- senna (or Senokot) one to four tablets at night

- bisacodyl 5–10 mg at night

- lactulose (for children) 2.5–5 ml twice daily

for long-term use (prevention)

- bran half to two tablespoonfuls/day

- ispaghula two tablespoon/day with plenty of water

- methylcellulose '450' three to six tablets twice daily with half
  pint of water

6 HIGH BLOOD PRESSURE

WHAT IS IT?

- **hypertension** is a 'mechanistic' diagnosis by sphygmomanometer when levels are above 160/95

- in majority (over 90%) it is **essential** (of uncertain cause) in the other 5–10% is **secondary**, e.g. kidney disease, endocrine disorders or effects of drugs (*note*: contraceptive pill)

grades of severity of GP cases in a practice of 2,500

	DBP	No. of cases (%)
Mild	90–109	320 (85%)
Moderate	110–129	50 (13·5%)
Severe	>130	5 (1·5%)
Total		375 (100%)

- most are **mild–moderate** and only few are **severe** or **malignant**

- importance and significance of high blood pressure are **possible preventable** complications:
    strokes (haemorrhagic)
    heart disease
    kidney failure
    retinopathy

WHO GETS IT AND WHEN?

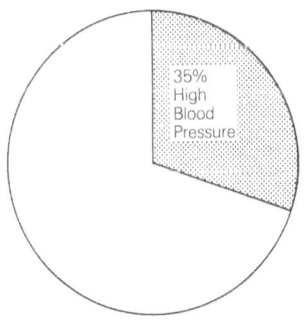

35% High Blood Pressure

- at any time 10–15% of the whole population has 'high blood pressure' (5–7 million in UK)

- one third of adults over 40 have high blood pressure

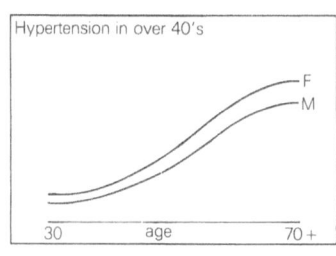

Hypertension in over 40's

- **prevalence** rises with age and is higher in females

Hypertension in population of 2500

New cases diagnosed (annual incidence)	12
In practice (prevalence)	375
age 30–64	225
age 65+	150

- in a **general practice** of 2500 there are 375 hypertensives

WHAT HAPPENS?

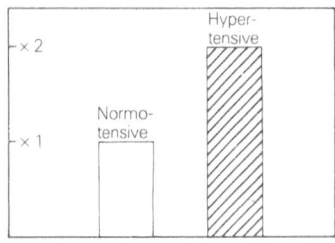

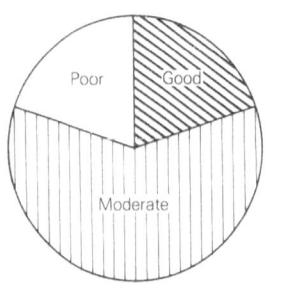

- high blood pressure (BP) doubles the **risk of premature death** (before 70) from
  strokes
  heart disease
- **extra risk factors**

> M > F
> age under 60 (at diagnosis)
> family history of early deaths from
>   stroke/heart disease
> smoking
> high levels of blood pressure
> + raised plasma lipids

- it is not easy with treatment to achieve good control of high blood pressure
  good control (DBP < 90 mm) in 20%
  moderate control (DBP 90–109 mm) in 60%
  poor control (DBP > 110 mm) in 20%

HIGH BLOOD PRESSURE

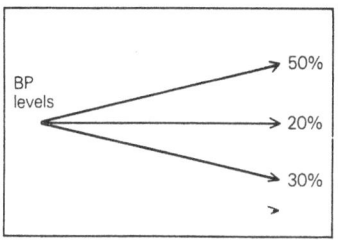

BP levels

50%

20%

30%

- do not assume that BP will inevitably rise with time – in half it may fall naturally or remain same without treatment
- because we do not know the exact causes and do not have specific treatments the extent of success in controlling high blood pressure is imperfect

---

HIGH BLOOD PRESSURE: A RECAP

- high prevalence with age
- most are 'essential' of uncertain cause for which there are no specific treatments
- overall it shortens life
- risk groups
  high levels of systolic BP and diastolic BP
  M > F
  under 60s
  smokers
  family history positive
- blood pressure may come down naturally in some individuals without treatment
- question is whether all or some hypertensives should be treated, and if so, which ones?

WHAT TREATMENT?

objectives

- decide whether a person with raised BP really needs long-term therapy
- decide on extra risk factors that influence decisions to treat
- to reduce BP to near 'normal' levels
- to avoid side effects of drugs
- advise on non-drug measures
- introduce a long-term programme of screening, early diagnosis and long-term supervision of hypertensives

DRUGS IN HYPERTENSION

- the height of the blood pressure is determined by the cardiac output and the total peripheral resistance
- in hypertension the major abnormality is an increase in peripheral resistance the cause of which is unknown
- drugs lower blood pressure by reducing peripheral resistance or lowering cardiac output or both
- ideally reducing peripheral resistance and leaving the normal vascular reflexes intact would be the best way of lowering blood pressure
- drugs which lower cardiac output, although effective, can compromise the peripheral circulation – this may not matter clinically but can cause problems particularly in the elderly (see beta-blockers)
- there is no ideal anti-hypertensive drug yet available

β-ADRENERGIC BLOCKERS

what are they and how do they work?

- competitive inhibition of β-adrenergic receptors
- selective blocks affect predominantly:
  selective β_1-receptors (heart)
  non-selective β_1- and β_2-receptors (heart, blood vessels and bronchi)
- lower both systolic and diastolic blood pressures without postural fall – not known how this is achieved
- prevent usual rise of pulse rate, cardiac output and cardiac work on exercise

effects

benefits

- β-blockers produce a significant fall in pressure in 50% of hypertensives

- bronchospasm facilitated
- do NOT use in asthmatics
- in wheezy bronchitics use a selective β-blocker
  (*note*: β-antagonists, such as salbutamol, reverse actions of β-blockers)

- exacerbate cardiac failure because of reduced sympathetic drive to the heart
- cause cold hands and feet and exacerbate peripheral vascular disease by reducing peripheral circulation
- suppress the warning signals of hypoglycaemia, so warn insulin-taking diabetics
- limited exercise tolerance due to reduced cardiac output
- many on therapy lack drive, energy and aggression
- impotence
- propranolol particularly liable to cause nightmares and depression

interactions

- do not give i.v. verapamil to patients on β-blockers – both depress cardiac function
- ergotamine increases peripheral vasoconstriction with β-blockers
- many NSAIA's reduce BP lowering effects of β-blockers

what available?

- large number of β-blockers available which differ in selectivity and duration of action
- a few are also partial agonists with a sympathetic stimulating action and maintain a higher resting pulse rate

Drug	Selectivity	Partial agonist	Half life (h)	Dose[a] (mg) Angina	Dose[a] (mg) Hypertension
Acebutalol	selective	+	8	200 bd to 300 tid	400 once to 400 tid
Atenolol	selective	–	8	50–200 once daily	50–200 once daily
Metoprolol	selective	–	3	50–100 bd or tds	100–200 bd or 200 slow release daily
Nadolol	non-selective	–	20	40–160 daily	80–240 daily
Oxprenolol	non-selective	+	2	40–80 tid	80–160 bd or 160 slow release
Pindolol	non-selective	+ +	4	5 bd or tid	15–30 once daily
Propranolol	non-selective	–	3	40–80 bd or tid 160 slow release	80–160 bd or 160 slow release
Sotalol	non-selective	–	12	80–200 bd	80–300 bd
Timolol	non-selective	–	5	5–15 tid	10 once to 20 tid

[a]Doses of β-blockers may require adjustment depending on individual responses.

which to use?

- choice is personal (by doctor)
- all are equally effective in lowering blood pressure
- **For example**: atenolol and metoprolol are selective, dosage is easy to adjust, central effects are rare while if resting pulse is low, oxprenolol is useful

how to use?

- **check history** of asthma, peripheral vascular disease and heart failure

- **For example**: start with atenolol 50 mg in morning
  metoprolol 200 mg (slow release) in morning
- fall in blood pressure may be slow so dose should be increased only at 2 week intervals
- with impaired renal function use metoprolol
- with impaired liver function use atenolol
- **labetalol** is a combined β-blocker and α-blocker (vasodilator)
    Dosage is difficult to adjust
    produces immediate fall in blood pressure
    100 mg b.d. increasing to 1·2 g b.d. if necessary, at 2 week intervals
    adverse effects as for β-blockers plus postural hypotension and tingling of scalp

DIURETICS

what are they and how do they work?

- thiazide diuretics are best
- cause hypovolaemia and fall in blood pressure
- hypovolaemia restored in succeeding months, but blood pressure lowering effect persists by direct action on arterioles

effects

benefits

- thiazides, acting alone, lower BP in 40%
- thiazides are useful in combination with β-blockers, vasodilators and ACE inhibitors

risks

- prolonged use may cause metabolic upsets
    - **diabetes**: usually reversible on stopping thiazide
    - **gout**: from uric acid retention
    - **hypokalaemia**: particularly with large doses
  - impotence (20%)
  - rashes (rare)

what available and how to use?

- there are many to choose from – here are selected examples

• bendrofluazide	2·5 mg
• cyclopenthiazide	0·25 mg
• polythiazide	0.5 mg
• **all given each morning**	

- low dosage minimizes metabolic complications without compromising efficiency
- loop diuretics only in patients with impaired renal function
- **plasma potassium** should be checked after 1 month – it is rarely below 3·0 mmol/l, but if it is, then add amiloride 5 mg daily and recheck plasma potassium

COMBINATIONS OF β-BLOCKERS AND DIURETIC

- most β-blockers are available combined with a thiazide as fixed ratio preparations
- may help in compliance and in forgetful patients
- *Note*: each drug will have its problems, particularly those preparations which also contain a potassium-sparing diuretic – with these preparations dangerous potassium retention may occur in renal failure

POTASSIUM-SPARING DIURETICS

what are they and how do they work?
- mild diuretics which do not cause potassium depletion
- **spironolactone** inhibits the effects of aldosterone on the kidney
- **amiloride** affects the distal tubule

effects

benefits
- hypotensive effect is similar to thiazides
- often combined with a thiazide

risks
- both can cause dangerous potassium retention with impaired renal function or excessive potassium intake
- spironolactone also causes
  nausea
  gynaecomastia and menstrual
    problems
  augments action of digoxin

when and how to use?
- only use when potassium loss is a problem (rare)
- spironolactone: 50–100 mg daily
- amiloride: 5–10 mg daily

VASODILATORS

what are they and how do they work?
- lower blood pressure by dilating arterioles

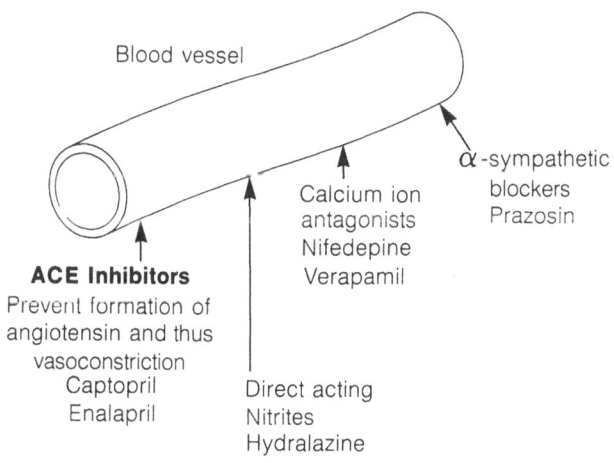

Blood vessel

α-sympathetic blockers
Prazosin

Calcium ion antagonists
Nifedepine
Verapamil

ACE Inhibitors
Prevent formation of angiotensin and thus vasoconstriction
Captopril
Enalapril

Direct acting
Nitrites
Hydralazine

Comparison of calcium channel blockers		
	nifedipine	*verapamil*
Heart muscle	—	negative inotrope
Heart conducting system	—	depressed
Coronary arteries	dilated	dilated
Arteries	dilated	dilated
Veins	dilated	dilated
Blood pressure	↓	↓

- **calcium channel blockers**
  slow the intake of calcium by cells
    nifedipine relaxes arterioles and
      coronary vessels
    verapamil has similar action and also
      depresses conduction in the AV node

- **hydralazine** acts as a direct arteriolar dilator

- **prazosin** dilates arterioles by α_1-sympathetic blockade

- **angiotensin-converting enzyme (ACE) inhibitors** prevent formation of angiotensin II which is a vasoconstrictor and which also causes aldosterone secretion. Available as:
    captopril
    enalapril

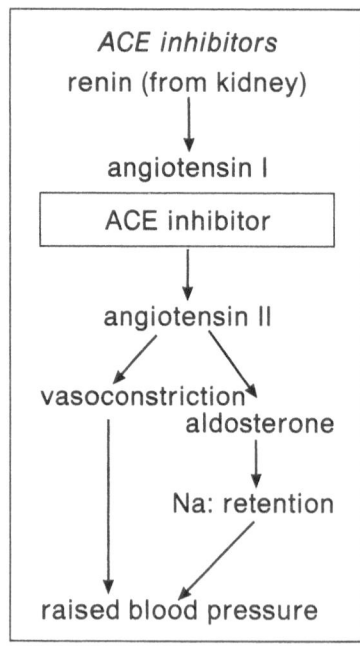

ACE inhibitors

renin (from kidney)
↓
angiotensin I

ACE inhibitor
↓
angiotensin II

vasoconstriction ↘ aldosterone
↓ ↓
Na: retention
↓ ↙
raised blood pressure

effects

benefits

- immediate fall in blood pressure which is largely non-postural

risks

- **calcium channel blockers**
  flushing and headache
  hot legs
  swelling of ankles with **nifedipine**
  occasional dyspepsia
  verapamil constipates

- **note**: injection of verapamil in patient on a beta-blocker is dangerous

- **hydralazine**
  flushing and headache
  tachycardia (combine with beta-blocker)
  higher doses (over 100 mg daily) associated with SLE-like syndrome
  genetic differences in rates of metabolism with variable toxicity and response

- **prazosin**
  profound fall in BP with first dose so start with 0·5 mg and give before retiring
  headache, nasal stuffiness and tiredness

- **ACE inhibitors**:   both **enalapril** and **captopril**
  severe hypotension with first dose, particularly if patient is on diuretic
  hyperkalaemia with potassium sparing diuretics or in renal failure
  monitor plasma potassium in this group

- **note**: patients starting any ACE inhibitors should be observed for 3 h after taking first dose because of possible sudden fall in blood pressure

- captopril
    severe proteinuria (> 3 g per 24 h) in
        1% neutropoenia in first 3 months of
        treatment in renal failure or SLE
    loss of taste – returns when drug is
        stopped
- **note**: provided the dose of captopril does
    not exceed 75 mg per 24 h, risk to fit
    hypertensives is low

which to use?

- **nifedipine** is easy to use but high rate of
    minor side effects (most cease with
    continued treatment)
- **verapamil**, cheap alternative to nifedipine
- **prazosin** is safe (providing that first dose
    hypotension is avoided), dose adjustment
    may be difficult
- **ACE inhibitors**, side effects rare but can
    be unpleasant, dose should be kept low

how to use?

- **nifedipine** (slow release)
    20 mg b.d. and increase if necessary
- **verapamil**
    120 mg b.d. and increase if necessary
    maximum dose: 480 mg in 24 h
- **prazosin**
    0·5 mg before retiring as first dose
    0·5 mg t.i.d. and increase slowly if
        necessary
    note: fall in BP may be marked if on
        other hypotensive drugs
- **captopril**
    6·25 mg b.d. and increase if necessary
        to maximum of 25 mg t.i.d.
    in high risk group (renal disease, SLE
        and immuno-suppressed) blood
        count every 2 weeks for 3 months and
        urine test for protein for 9 months

- **enalapril**
  5 mg once daily increasing to
  20 mg daily if necessary

- **note**: severe hypotension may occur in patients on thiazides on first receiving ACE inhibitors
- **note**: if ACE inhibitor fails, add thiazide and NOT a β-blocker
- **note**:start with half dose in the elderly

TREATMENT PLAN

note:
- hypertension *per se* is not a 'disease' but a body feature that leads to premature death and disability and increases risks of stroke, heart failure, myocardial infarction and rarely of renal failure and serious retinopathy
- aims of treatment are to diagnose hypertension early and to control it to prevent complications if considered likely to develop
- early diagnosis is responsibility of general practitioner through opportunistic or planned screening exercises
- since decision to treat is probably long term, make sure that diagnosis is correct before starting, and that risks of morbidity outweigh disturbance to patient and costs of treatment. Unless urgent indications take at least three separate readings at weekly intervals
- planned long-term care by same physician is best

urgent reduction of blood pressure is required:
- in hypertensive encephalopathy, e.g. headache, fits, papilloedema and retinopathy, BP > 230/130
- in dissecting aortic aneurysm
- in very high diastolic BP > 140 mmHg
- this is best achieved in hospital with monitoring
- *In an emergency*:
  hydralazine 10 mg i.m. four hourly, *or*
  nifedipine 10 mg capsule cut open and contents held in mouth
  (do NOT lower blood pressure too rapidly because of danger of cerebrovascular ischaemia)

fairly urgent reduction of blood pressure is required:
- when blood pressure is > 220/120 (on more than a single reading)
- retinopathy and/or left ventricular hypertrophy present
- risk factors present when patient is:
  male
  under 60
  family history of early cardiovascular deaths
- start with *β-blockers*:
  atenolol 50–100 mg once daily
  review in 2 weeks

- if response inadequate (BP > 190/110); *add vasodilator*
    - nifedipine retard 20 mg twice daily *or* hydralazine *or* prazosin
- if control still poor (BP > 190/110):
    add diuretic
    - bendrofluazide 2·5–5 mg daily

non-urgent (mild-moderate hypertension)

- blood pressure initially 160/95 to 200/109

- no evidence of cardiovascular complications

- it is justifiable to wait for a few months with *general advice* (stop smoking, reduce alcohol, reduce weight, reduce salt intake) and to recheck blood pressure

- if drug therapy decided upon, adopt step-by-step policy – this may take 1–2 months for full response to be apparent

- start with *diuretic*
    bendrofluazide 2·5 mg daily, *or*
    β-blocker
    atenolol 50–100 mg daily

- if response inadequate (BP > 170/100):
    combine diuretic and *β*-blocker

- if response still inadequate (BP > 170/100):
    combine diuretic and *β*-blocker and vasodilator
    nifedipine, hydralazine or prazosin

- aim to reduce blood pressure to < 150/95

- *note*: in this mild-moderate group treatment results in a 20% reduction in cardiovascular events and strokes: this represents only 1.6 events per 1000 patient treatment years – therefore need for careful consideration before long-term therapy is justified in patient (45–60) with hypertension at lower end of range

elderly (> 60 years)

- only treat if blood pressure is persistently > 200/105 and/or cardiovascular complications

- *β*-blockers are less effective and side effects more troublesome in this group

- start with *diuretic*
    bendrofluazide 2·5 mg daily

- if response inadequate (BP > 180/100): consider adding:
  vasodilator
     nifedipine retard 20 mg twice daily (may be too much)
- *note*: treatment in this group results in only a 25% reduction in cardiovascular events and strokes representing 29 events per 1000 treatment years (or 11 strokes per 1000 treatment years) – consider carefully before starting long-term treatment

alternative regimes

quality of life is important in long-term treatment; there may be many side effects of the drugs used that may be unacceptable to some patients, particularly with β-blockers; a different regime can be adopted.

- start with *ACE inhibitor*:
     captopril 6·25 mg twice daily, *or*
     enalapril 5 mg daily
     increase both as necessary
- if this fails to control blood pressure: *add*
  diuretic
     bendrofluazide 2·5–5 mg daily, *or*
  vasodilator
     nifedipine retard 20 mg twice daily
     (verapamil may be more acceptable)

note: in all patients who fail to respond as expected:

- check for compliance
- check that other drugs are not being taken that may reverse the anti-hypertensive actions, e.g. NSAIAs
- even with treatment it may be difficult to achieve good results
- a balance has to be struck between enjoying life with raised blood pressure and lowering the blood pressure with concomitant unpleasant side-effects from the drugs used.

7   ANGINA

WHAT IS IT?

- a feature of the clinical ischaemic heart disease syndrome (IHD)
- produced by **temporary functional ischaemia of the myocardium** resulting from
  - increased demand
  - transient arterial spasm
    - or fixed partial occlusion

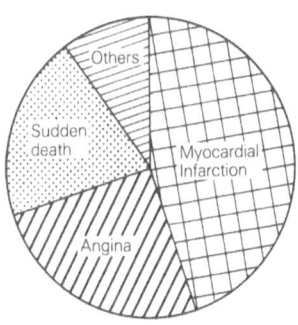

pathophysiology

- arteriosclerotic occlusion of coronary arteries
- poor correlation between clinical picture and angiography
- ECG is normal in 50% of those with angina

risk factors

- smoking
- high blood cholesterol and/or triglycerides
- high blood pressure
- diabetes
- obesity
- contraceptive pill
- **family history** of IHD or sudden death

angina may be triggered by

- anaemia
- thyroid disease ('hypo' more than 'hyper')
- aortic valve disease

WHO GETS IT AND WHEN?

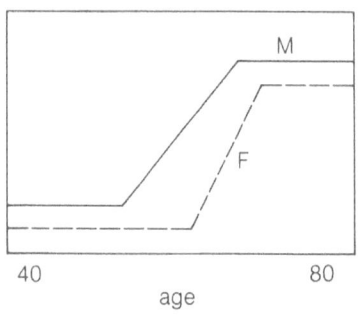

- a condition of *ageing*
- M > F in under 60s
- F = M in over 60s

angina	
New cases	4
Persons consulting with angina	25
all IHD	
New cases	15
Persons consulting with IHD	70

- **annual prevalence** in a general practice of 2500

WHAT HAPPENS?

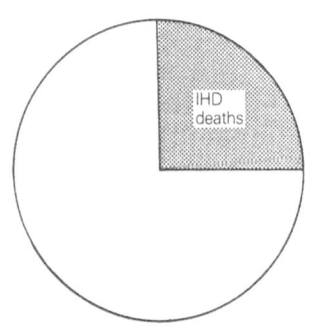

- IHD is largest single cause of death
- 25% of all IHD deaths are in over 65s
- 40% of premature deaths in males 45–60 are from IHD

70

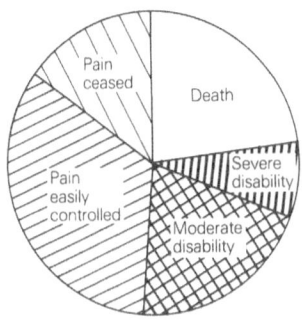

- five-year follow-up of angina

death	23%
severe angina (uncontrolled)	8%
moderate (disabling but controllable)	20%
mild (inconvenient)	35%
cessation of symptoms	14%

prognostic factors

Annual mortality	
1 vessel disease	1–2%
2 vessel disease	6%
3 vessel disease	10%
L. main vessel	20%
'stable angina'	4%
'unstable angina' (in first year)	17%

surgery

Results of surgery	
angina ceases at 1 year	80%
angina-free at 5 years	50%
mortality of surgery	1–2%

- probably for about 10% of angina patients in failed medical treatment and in unstable angina
- coronary artery by-pass graft or angioplasty

ANGINA: A RECAP
- part of IHD syndrome
- a frequent clinical condition
- controllable risk factors
- after 5 years one third are dead or severely disabled

WHAT TREATMENT?

objectives
- to relieve symptoms
- to improve function
- to prevent complications:
  sudden death
  myocardial infarction
  arrhythmias
  heart failure
- to prolong useful life

DRUGS

NITRATES

what are they and how do they work?
- organic nitrates and nitrites and inorganic nitrates act directly as smooth muscle relaxants

ACTION OF DRUGS USED IN ANGINA

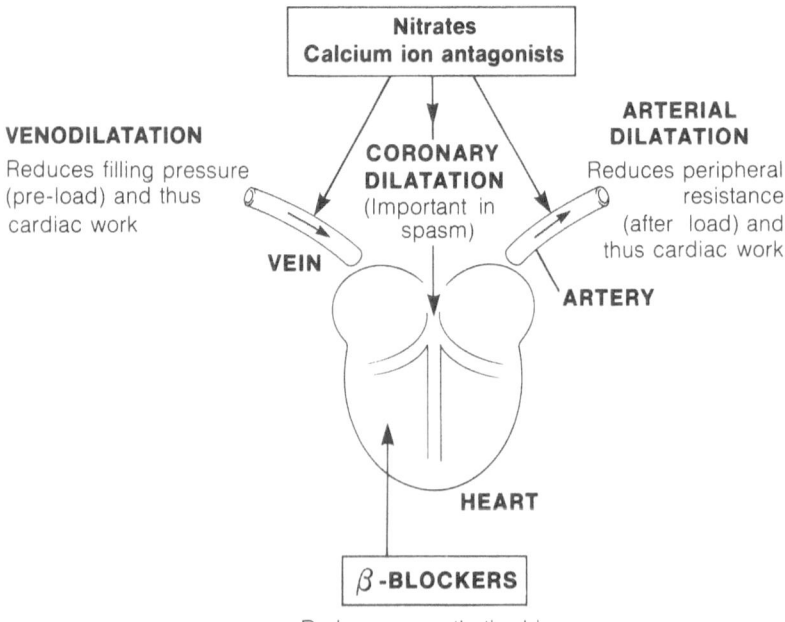

Nitrates
Calcium ion antagonists

VENODILATATION
Reduces filling pressure (pre-load) and thus cardiac work

CORONARY DILATATION
(Important in spasm)

ARTERIAL DILATATION
Reduces peripheral resistance (after load) and thus cardiac work

VEIN

ARTERY

HEART

β-BLOCKERS

Reduce sympathetic drive and thus cardiac work

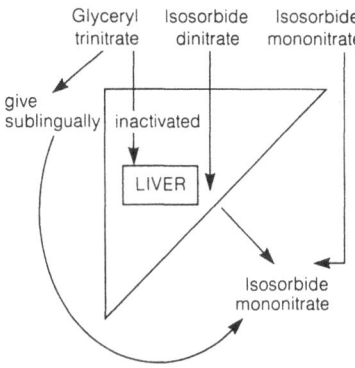

- they dilate veins and arteries leading to peripheral pooling of blood with a reduction of venous return to the heart and reduction of cardiac work and oxygen requirements
- peripheral resistance and blood pressure fall
- coronary vasodilatation is of doubtful therapeutic significance, unless spasm is a factor
- **glyceryl trinitrate** is inactivated in the liver if swallowed and acts only through absorption from mouth after sucking or chewing
- **isosorbide dinitrate** is broken down in liver to the active mononitrate

effects

benefits

- relief of anginal pain and better anticipatory prevention of angina

	Onset of effect	Duration of effect
Glyceryl trinitrate (suck/chew)	2 min	30 min
Isosorbide dinitrate (chewed) (swallowed)	2 min 10 min	2 h 5 h
Isosorbide mononitrate (swallowed)	20 min	10 h

risks

- headaches, short duration if dose low
- flushing, hypotension (fainting), probably decrease with continued use
- *note:* do NOT use in anaemia and glaucoma

which to use?

acute attack

- glyceryl trinitrate
- isosorbide dinitrate (chewed)

prevention

- isosorbide mononitrate
- isosorbide dinitrate

how to use?

- **glyceryl trinitrate** tablets, 0.5 mg per dose
  chew or suck when necessary and spit
  out or swallow when pain relieved
  repeat as often as necessary
  unstable, so discard after 8 weeks
- **isosorbide mononitrate,** 20 mg
  two or three times a day to maximum of
  120 mg daily, orally for prevention
- **isosorbide dinitrate** chewable tablets
  5 mg for immediate effect
  tablets 10–20 mg four to six hourly orally
  for prevention
- warn patients of likely side-effects but
  reassure that they will decrease with time

CALCIUM CHANNEL ANTAGONISTS

**what are they and how do
they work? (see also
p. 62)**

- relax smooth muscle of arterioles and
  veins producing vasodilatation and
  decrease in cardiac work
- direct action on coronary arteries may be
  important in spasm

effects

benefits

- prevention of angina
- nifedipine relieves attack in 5 min if held in
  mouth

risks

(see pp. 63 in section on hypertension)

what available?

- nifedipine
- verapamil
- diltiazem

ANGINA

which to use?	• all three effective
	• verapamil has anti-arrhythmic action and negative inotropic effect
how to use?	• *nifedipine:* 10 mg
	for **attack** cut capsule with knife (tough) and empty contents into mouth for quick relief
	for **prevention** three times daily (half dose for elderly)
	• *verapamil:* 80 mg three times daily and increase if necessary to 120 mg three times daily
	• *diltiazem:* 60 mg three times daily (twice daily in elderly or with impaired liver and kidney function) and increased if necessary to 360 mg daily

β-BLOCKERS

what are they and how do they work?	• competitive inhibition of β-adrenergic receptors
	• prevent increase of cardiac work and oxygen consumption with exercise and other forms of sympathetic stimulation

effects

benefits	• provide continuous prophylactic prevention of anginal attacks
risks	(see Chapter 6 on hypertension)
	• do NOT use in patients with asthma and heart failure
	• care in patients with peripheral vascular disease and diabetics on insulin

- do NOT stop β-blockers suddenly as may precipitate arrhythmia, angina or infarction; withdraw stepwise
- ineffective if coronary spasm a feature

which to use?

- choice of β-blocker is a personal one (see below)
- β-blockade must be maintained continuously

how to use?

- lower but more frequent dosage than for hypertension
- timing of dosage tailored to prevention of angina
- *atenolol* 50–100 mg once daily
- *metoprolol* 50–100 mg three times daily
- *propranolol* 40 mg three times daily, increase if necessary

TREATMENT PLAN

note:
- angina is a symptom complex that is caused by relative and transient myocardial ischaemia from coronary artery narrowing
- treatment aims to improve coronary artery circulation and reduce myocardial oxygen demand and work of the heart
- drug treatment relieves but cannot cure the occlusion by the sclerotic coronary arteries, only by-pass grafts with veins from legs or angioplasty can do this
- in a few patients coronary artery spasm may cause symptoms

general measures
- stop smoking
- reduce excessive weight by diet
- control raised blood pressure
- correct possible causes such as anaemia and high blood cholesterol
- alter lifestyle and habits to avoid attacks

drugs

acute attack
- glyceryl trinitrate 0.5 mg suck or dissolve sublingually, *or*
- isosorbide dinitrate 5 mg chew and keep in mouth (relief of pain should occur within 2–5 min)

Prevention of attack
- with infrequent attacks and recognized precipitant: glyceryl trinitrate to be sucked *before* engaging in activities likely to cause an attack
- with more frequent attacks: *add beta-blockers* on a regular basis
  atenolol 50–100 mg daily, *or*
  propranolol 40–320 mg daily
- if attacks not controlled *add:*
  isosorbide mononitrate 20–80 mg daily, *or*
  isosorbide dinitrate 20–120 mg daily on a regular basis, *or*
  nifedipine 20–60 mg daily
- if *spasm* is considered a factor (irregular pattern of pain and attacks of pain at rest):
  nitrates and/or
  nifedipine
  do NOT use β-blockers

- if *unstable angina* present (prolonged pain not relieved by trinitrate and unchanged ECG):
    bed rest
    isosorbide mononitrate 20 mg three times daily
    nifedipine 5–10 mg three times daily
    β-blockers if tachycardia

surgery

- to be considered if angina is not controlled with drugs and general measures
- also in increasing and recent onset of unstable angina

note:

- in majority (two thirds) of persons with angina, symptoms can be controlled with medication
- surgery will be necessary only in about 10% of all angina cases
- whatever is done one quarter will die within 5 years

8 HEART FAILURE

WHAT IS IT?

- a clinical syndrome where heart fails to pump blood efficiently resulting in **backward** congestion of lungs and other organs and tissues and **forward** deprivation of blood supply
- two clinical types recognized **acute** and **chronic**

acute heart failure

- severe and sudden effects from acute reduction predominantly in output of left ventricle with pulmonary oedema
- predisposing causes are:
  high blood pressure
  ischaemic heart disease
  aortic valve disease
  mitral valve incompetence

chronic heart failure

- slower in onset and progressive with peripheral oedema as main feature and reduced cardiac output with impaired renal perfusion
- predisposing causes are:
  pulmonary disease
  mitral stenosis
  thyrotoxicosis
  cardiomyopathy
  secondary to left ventricular failure
- **note:** in many instances there is combined left and right cardiac failure

pathophysiology

- **L. ventricular hypertrophy and/or dilatation** lead to reduced cardiac output
- **homeostatic reflexes** attempt to maintain blood pressure
  sympathetic activation +
  $\longrightarrow$ tachycardia
  $\longrightarrow$ contractility
  $\longrightarrow$ vasoconstriction
  angiotensin release
  $\longrightarrow$ fluid retention
  $\longrightarrow$ vasoconstriction
  but increase strain on failing heart

who gets it and when?

- **annual prevalence** in a general practice of 2500

Heart failure – annual prevalence per 2500

Disease	Male	Female	Persons
Congestive heart failure	12	18	15
Left ventricular failure	2	2	2
Cor pulmonale	3	1	2
Cardiac arrhythmias	6	7	7
Total	23	28	26

WHAT HAPPENS?

acute left ventricular failure

- carries a high mortality rate if not treated quickly and appropriately
- once survived the future outlook depends on the underlying causal conditions

chronic heart failure

- if untreated life expectancy is 1–3 years
- with good response to therapy life expectancy may be improved

HEART FAILURE: A RECAP

- acute and chronic types
- acute is L. ventricular failure
- chronic is R. heart failure or mixture of R. and L. failure
- although end-product of many and varied diseases good opportunities for control
- outcomes depend on causal condition and on state of heart muscle

WHAT TREATMENT?

objectives

- control acute pulmonary oedema
- improve cardiac function and output
- reduce raised diastolic filling pressure and relieve pulmonary congestion
- reduce peripheral resistance
- whenever possible, correct underlying cause

**Diuretics and Vasodilators
in Heart Failure**

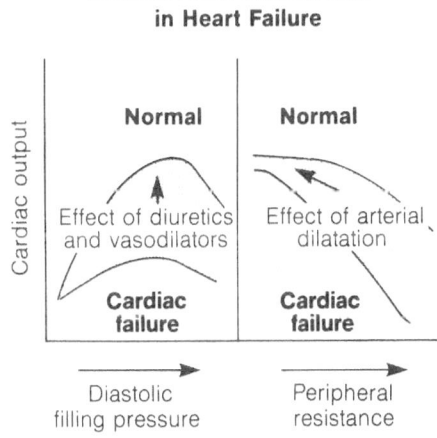

DRUGS

THIAZIDE DIURETICS

Proximal tubule   Distal tubule

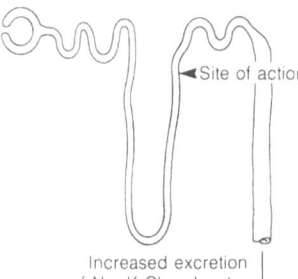

◄Site of action

Increased excretion
of Na, K Cl and water
up to 5 - 10% of filtered Na ▼

LOOP DIURETICS

Proximal tubule   Distal tubule

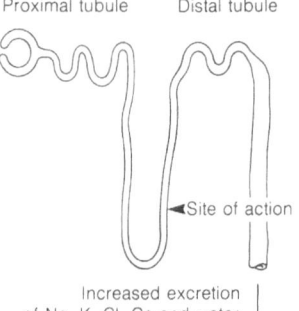

◄Site of action

Increased excretion
of Na, K, Cl, Ca and water
up to 15 - 20% of filtered Na ▼

AMILORIDE/SPIRONOLACTONE

Proximal tubule   Distal tubule

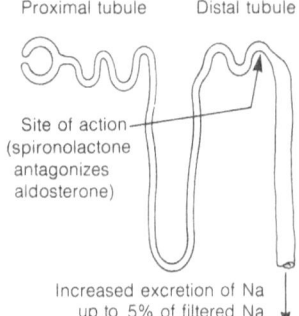

Site of action
(spironolactone
antagonizes
aldosterone)

Increased excretion of Na
up to 5% of filtered Na ▼

THIAZIDE DIURETICS

what are they and how do they work?
- prevent reabsorption of sodium and water and increase secretion of potassium by the renal tubule
- several are available with similar degrees of efficacy

effects

benefits
- moderate diuresis of varying duration which is only slightly dose-related (Also used in hypertension – see Chapter 6)

risks
- hypokalaemia which is dose-related
- uric acid retention causing gout
- reduced glucose tolerance with prolonged use – good diabetic control becomes difficult
- causes lithium retention
- NSAIAs reduce diuretic effects

what available and which to choose?
• there is no 'best buy' – therefore choose the cheapest

Drug	Duration of action (h)	Diuretic dose (daily)
Chlorothiazide	10	500 mg to 1 g
Hydrochlorothiazide	10	25–100 mg
Clopamide	15	20–60 mg
Bendrofluazide	20	5–10 mg
Hydroflumethiazide	15	25–200 mg
Polythiazide	24	1–4 mg
Cyclopenthiazide	12	250 μg to 1.0 mg
Chlorthalidone	48	50–200 mg (alt. days)

how to use?

• single daily dose in morning modified by patient response

• measure plasma creatinine and electrolytes before starting and after 1 month

• patients on low dose thiazides, full diet and no complicating factors rarely develop hypokalaemia (<3.2 mmol/l)

• the best way of judging diuretic efficacy is by weighing – so weigh at each consultation

• for patients at risk from hypokalaemia see below

LOOP DIURETICS

what are they and how do they work?
• frusemide and bumetanide are similar

• powerful inhibitors of sodium and potassium reabsorption together with water in the ascending limb of the renal tubule

effects

benefits
• dose-related diuresis

	• rapid action in 10 min, i.v., lasting 2 h; in 30 min, oral, lasting 6 h

risks
- hypokalaemia (see below)
- uric acid retention causing gout
- diabetic-like state
- deafness (may be permanent) more likely if given i.v. rapidly with aminoglycosides
- hypovolaemia with large diuresis
- bumetanide may cause myalgic and abdominal discomfort
- interacts with lithium and NSAIAs

which and how to use?

acute heart failure
- frusemide 20–60 mg slowly i.v. or i.m.
- bumetanide 1–2 mg slowly i.v. or i.m.

chronic heart failure
- frusemide 20–120 mg once daily orally time of administration must be adjusted to patient's life routine 80 mg twice daily in resistant cases
- bumetanide 1–2 mg daily

the problem of potassium
- thiazide and loop diuretics can cause hypokalaemia

at-risk patients
- high dosage of diuretics
- poor deficient diet
- elderly
- concurrent steroids
- those taking digitalis (increased risk of toxicity) or with arrhythmias
- nephrotic and cirrhotic patients

- give supplementary potassium (20–50 mmol required daily)
- potassium chloride SR (Slow-K) 8 mmol K per tablet
- effervescent potassium tablets (Sando-K) 12 mmol K per tablet
- potassium chloride syrup (Kay-Cee-L) 5 mmol K per 5 ml
- **note**: diuretics with added potassium supplements provide inadequate replacements **or**
- combine with potassium-sparing diuretic
- **note**: do NOT combine supplementary potassium with potassium-sparing diuretic – may lead to hyperkalaemia

POTASSIUM-SPARING DIURETICS

what are they and how do they work?

- amiloride and triamterene prevent sodium reabsorption in the distal renal tubule
- spironolactone antagonizes the action of aldosterone on the tubule and thus decreases sodium reabsorption

effects

benefits

- moderate diuretic action without excessive potassium loss and also reduces potassium loss due to other diuretics

risks

- hyperkalaemia – do not use with supplementary potassium, ACE inhibitors or with impaired renal function (particularly diabetics)
- spironolactone may also cause nausea, gynaecomastia, hirsutism and menstrual irregularities
- there are a number of **fixed combinations** available and in these the risks are those of both diuretics

what is available?

- single diuretic

amiloride	5 mg tablet
triamterene	50 mg tablet
spironolactone	25–50 mg or 100 mg tablets

- fixed combinations

Moduretic (amiloride
5 mg + hydrochlorothiazide 50 mg)

Dyazide (triamterene
50 mg + hydrochlorothiazide 25 mg)

Frumil (amiloride 5 mg + frusemide
40 mg)

Aldactide '25/50' (spironolactone
25/50 mg + hydroflumethiazide
25/50 mg)

which to use and how?

high risk

- patients at high risk of potassium depletion
- patients already with plasma potassium <3.2 mmol/l
- give amiloride 5 mg added to a thiazide or a loop diuretic
- plasma electrolytes and creatinine should be estimated before starting and after 1 month
- Moduretic and Frumil may assist compliance

elderly

- electrolyte disturbances are a serious risk
- give Dyazide one or two tablets daily, *or* Aldactide 25, two to four tablets daily

DIGITALIS

what is it and how does it work?
- cardiac glycoside which depresses conduction in the bundle of His and has some positive inotropic action on the ventricles (increases force of ventricular contraction)

effects

benefits
- slows ventricular rate in atrial fibrillation with improved cardiac function
- transient positive inotropic effect, but improvement minimal for a few weeks only
- lowers ventricular rate, and may reverse supraventricular tachycardia and atrial flutter

risks
- low therapeutic ratio
- toxicity includes various arrhythmias, nausea, vomiting and diarrhoea
- confusion in the elderly and disturbances of colour vision
- toxicity enhanced by poor renal function, especially in elderly, and by hypokalaemia
- action increased by spironolactone, verapamil and carbenoxolone
- avoid in Wolff–Parkinson–White syndrome, may exacerbate tachycardia

what is available?

> digoxin 62.5, 125 and 250 μg tablets
> 250 μg in 1 ml for injection

how to use?
- most effective in controlling rapid atrial fibrillation, with or without heart failure

- 500 μg (250 μg in elderly) followed by 250 μg (125 μg in elderly) eight hourly for 3 doses and then 125–250 μg (62.5 μg in elderly) daily for maintenance according to response
- can be given by i.v. injection of 250 μg repeated after 2 h – this is rarely necessary, best avoided and never given to patients already on oral digoxin
- plasma digoxin levels (0.9–2.0 ng/ml) for checking compliance or toxicity

POSITIVE INOTROPIC AGENTS

what are they and how do they work?
- ventricular muscle stimulants
- dopamine and dobutamine
- increase contractility of heart and thus raise output
- dopamine in low doses is also a renal vasodilator

effects

benefits
- raise cardiac output and blood pressure in severe hypotension after cardiac infarction and heart surgery
- use is highly specialized

VASODILATORS

what are they and how do they work?
- mixed group of arterial and venous vasodilators
- reduce peripheral resistance (after-load) and venous filling pressure (pre-load)
- this promotes better cardiac function

HEART FAILURE

TREATMENT PLAN

note:

- heart failure is failure of the heart pump with *backward* congestion of lungs and other organs and *forward* deprivation of a blood supply
- treat remediable cause if possible

acute left ventricular failure

aim: to control pulmonary oedema – high mortality if not controlled quickly

immediate

- sit up
- give oxygen (if available) by mask or nasal catheter at 4–6 l/min
- frusemide, i.v., 40 mg slowly, *or*
- bumetanide, i.v., 1–2 mg slowly

if dyspnoea and distress

- *add* morphine i.v. 5–10 mg + cyclizine 50 mg (patient with COAD 2.5 mg only)

if much bronchospasm

- aminophylline i.v. 200 mg slowly (but NOT if patient taking oral aminophylline)

if no quick response

- ADMIT TO INTENSIVE CARE

chronic heart failure

aims: to improve cardiac function and output by reducing raised ventricular filling pressure and to relieve pulmonary congestion – good prognosis with treatment

diuretics

- blood urea and electrolytes should be checked before treatment and after 1 month
- frusemide 20–120 mg daily, *or*
- bumetamide 1–2 mg daily

(hypokalaemia unlikely with full diet and low dose of diuretic)

for at-risk patients

- *add* Slow K or combine with amiloride 5 mg daily

in mild heart failure

- thiazide diuretic alone or with amiloride (or spironolactone or Dyazide in elderly) for patients at risk from hypokalaemia

digitalis

- main indication is to control fast atrial fibrillation
- digoxin 500 μg (250 μg in elderly) as starter
- digoxin 62.5–250 μg daily for maintenance

vasodilators

- in patients resistant to diuretics
- in view of possible side effects initial therapy must be under close supervision
- isosorbide dinitrate 30–120 mg daily, *or*
- hydralazine 25–200 mg daily, *or (most effective)*
- ACE inhibitor captopril 12.5–75 mg daily with careful monitoring

9 CARDIAC ARRHYTHMIAS

WHAT ARE THEY?

- any disturbance of the heart's rhythm is a cardiac arrhythmia
- may range from symptoms of anxiety to sudden death
- may have cardiac or non-specific causes
- **cardiac**
  ischaemic heart disease
  cardiomyopathy
  mitral stenosis
  high blood presssure
  mitral valve prolapse
  Wolff–Parkinson–White syndrome

- **non-cardiac**
  anxiety
  coffee, alcohol
  thyroid disease
  drugs
  smoking
  carcinoma of bronchus

- **classification** (rate)
  tachycardias (> 100 beats/min)
  bradycardias (< 60 beats/min)

site of origin

- **sinus**
  tachycardia
  bradycardia

- **supraventricular**
  atria: flutter
              fibrillation
  AV node: ectopics
                 tachycardia

- **ventricular**
  - ectopics
  - tachycardia

- **conducting system**
  - AV heart blocks

diagnosis
- history and physical examination rarely help
- precise diagnosis only possible by ECG
- in presence of the arrhythmia, this may require long-term monitoring

significance
- the outcome depends on the underlying cause and the nature of the arrhythmia

ventricular tachycardia
- usually indicates serious underlying heart disease
  often complicates acute myocardial infarction

ventricular ectopics
- usually, but not always, benign
- remember alcohol, coffee and smoking as causes

supraventricular ectopics and tachycardia
- not usually associated with heart disease
- tachycardia can be a worrying nuisance

atrial flutter
- usually but not inevitably due to heart disease

atrial fibrillation
- often due to heart disease but may be 'lone' unassociated with cardiac disease

- remember alcohol and thyroxicosis as possible causes

congenital AV block

- good prognosis

bundle branch block

- variable significance
- minor degrees rarely important

WHO GETS THEM WHEN?

- arrhythmias are frequent

Annual prevalence of cardiac arrhythmics in a population of 2500	
Sinus tachycardia	20
Supraventricular ectopics	15
Supraventricular tachycardia	5
Atrial fibrillation	10
Atrial flutter	<1
Ventricular ectopics	10
Ventricular tachycardia	?
Sinus bradycardia	7
Heart block	5
(AV and BBB)	

age incidence

- they can occur at all ages

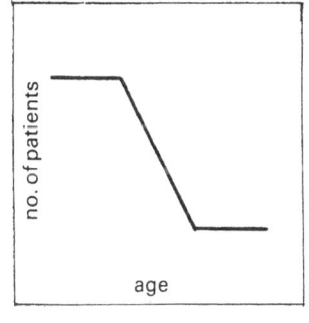

- sinus tachycardia (physiological)
- sinus bradycardia (physiological)
- Wolff–Parkinson–White syndrome

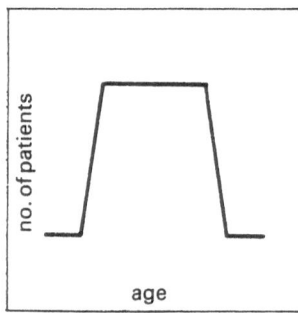

- thyroid disease
- alcoholism
- mitral stenosis
- IHD

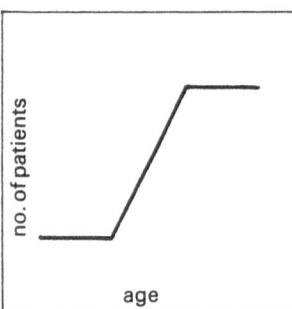

- high blood pressure
- myocardial infarction
- IHD
- iatrogenic (drug effects)
- heart block

WHAT TREATMENT?

objectives

- terminate or control arrhythmia during attack
- eliminate precipitating causes
- prevent recurrence
- monitor for side-effects of drugs

ANTI-ARRHYTHMIC DRUGS

what are they and how do they work?

classification   • is not easy

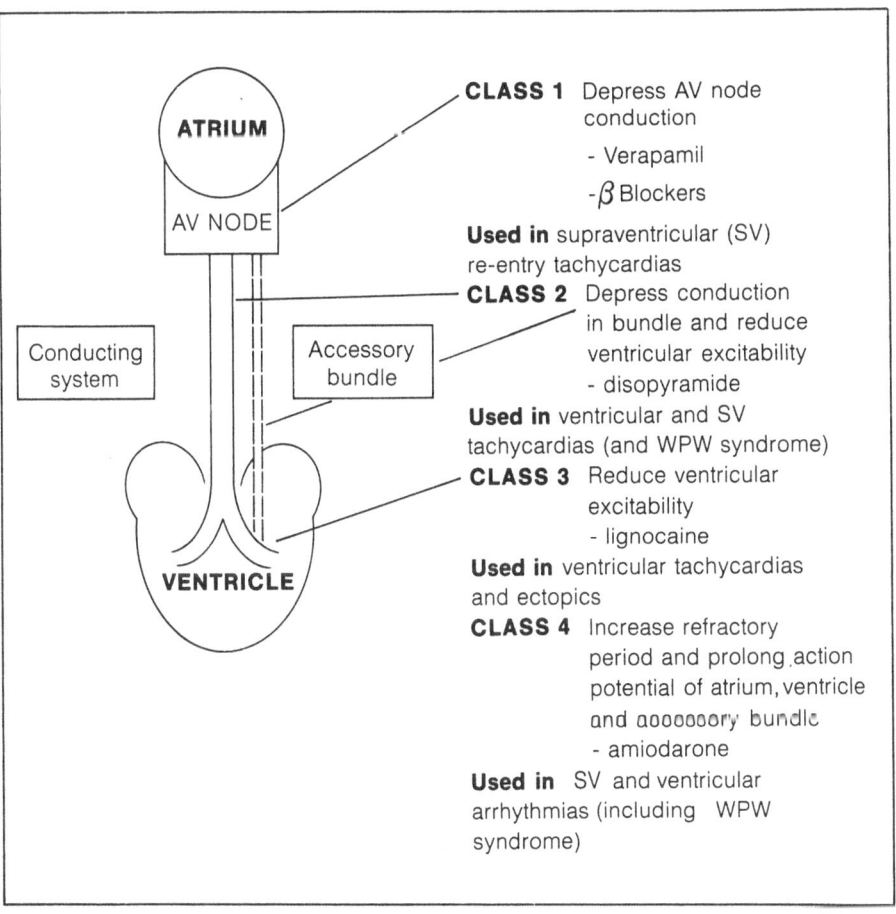

CLASS 1 Depress AV node
conduction
- Verapamil
- β Blockers

Used in supraventricular (SV)
re-entry tachycardias

CLASS 2 Depress conduction
in bundle and reduce
ventricular excitability
- disopyramide

Used in ventricular and SV
tachycardias (and WPW syndrome)

CLASS 3 Reduce ventricular
excitability
- lignocaine

Used in ventricular tachycardias
and ectopics

CLASS 4 Increase refractory
period and prolong action
potential of atrium, ventricle
and accessory bundle
- amiodarone

Used in SV and ventricular
arrhythmias (including WPW
syndrome)

Atrium, AV NODE, Conducting system, Accessory bundle, VENTRICLE

note:

• intravenous use of anti-arrhythmic drugs
to terminate an attack should only be
carried out with monitoring

• anti-arrhythmic drugs are more effective if
plasma potassium level is > 4.0 mmol/l

VERAPAMIL

what is it and how does it work?
- calcium channel antagonist
- depresses conduction in AV node and reverts SV arrhythmias due to re-entry phenomena
- also vasodilator and lowers blood pressure

effects

benefits
- reversion of SV arrhythmias (including those associated with Wolff–Parkinson–White syndrome)
- most useful drug for this purpose

risks
- negative inotrope – must not be given i.v. to patients on beta-blockers, will cause excessive cardiac depression
- potentiates action of digoxin (see p. 87)

how to use?

to revert an attack
- verapamil 5–10 mg i.v. over 2 min – if this fails, a further 5 mg can be given after 5 min

to prevent attacks
- verapamil 40–120 mg three times daily

DISOPYRAMIDE

what is it and how does it work?
- membrane stabiliser
- decreases ventricular excitability
- depresses conduction in accessory bundle
- anticholinergic

effects

benefits

- **given i.v.** terminates attack of both SV and ventricular tachycardias
- **given orally** prevents recurrent attacks

risks

- powerful negative inotrope can cause hypotension
- given to some types of SVT, particularly flutter or with narrow QRS, can cause a 'paradoxical' rise in ventricular rate
- do NOT use in cardiac failure and conduction defects
- can cause nausea, dry mouth, urinary retention, glaucoma and paralysis of accommodation (anti-cholinergic effects)

how to give?

to terminate attack

- best avoided in SVT unless there is precise information on its nature
- only give under ECG monitoring with facilities for resuscitation
- disopyramide 2 mg/kg i.v. over 5 min (maximum 150 mg)

to prevent attacks of ventricular ectopics or tachycardia

- disopyramide tablet 100 mg three times daily initially and increased, if necessary, to 200 mg three times daily, or sustained release 250–375 mg twice daily

LIGNOCAINE

what is it and how does it work?

- membrane stabilizing drug which reduces ventricular excitability
- metabolized in liver – large first pass effect

effects

benefits
- terminates attacks of ventricular arrhythmias

risks
- negative inotrope and may lower BP
- do NOT use with conduction defects
- reduce dose in heart failure (because of poor liver perfusion) or liver disease
- if dose too high – tremor and fits

how to give?
- given to terminate ventricular tachycardia or multiple ectopics
- lignocaine 100 mg bolus i.v. injection over 1 min followed by infusion at 4.0 mg/min reducing over next hour to minimal suppressive dose (1–2 mg/min)
- with impaired liver function infusion should not exceed 1.0 mg/min

AMIODARONE

what is it and how does it work?
- prolongs refractory period and action potential of atrium, ventricle and depresses conduction
- very long half-life of 28 days

effects

benefits
- effective for ventricular and SV arrhythmias (including Wolff–Parkinson–White syndrome) to terminate and prevent attacks
- weak negative inotrope

risks
- do NOT use in conduction defects

- corneal micro-deposits may cause haloes, disappear when drug stopped
- photosensitivity and grey pigmentation of skin
- hyper- or hypo-thyroidism
- pulmonary fibrosis
- peripheral neuropathy – irreversible
- hepatitis
- potentiates action of digoxin
- risks too high for routine use

how to give?

to prevent attacks
- amiodarone 200 mg three times daily for 1 week then 200 mg daily and reduce to minimum dose

to terminate attack
- amiodarone 5 mg/kg in 250 ml of 5% dextrose given over 30 min via central line to avoid thrombosis
- rapid infusion may cause severe hypotension

β-BLOCKERS

what are they and how do they work?
- depress conduction in AV node (see also chapter 6)

effcots

benefits
- prevention of SV tachycardia

risks
- negative inotrope
- do not combine with i.v. verapamil

| **how to use?** | • atenolol 50–100 mg orally once daily |
| | • may be combined cautiously with digoxin to increase control of ventricular rate in atrial fibrillation |

DIGOXIN

| **what is it and how does it work?** | • depresses conduction in AV node |

effects

benefits	• termination and prevention of attacks of SV tachycardia
	• control of ventricular rate in atrial fibrillation
	• control of ventricular rate or termination or conversion to atrial fibrillation in atrial flutter
risks	• must not be used in SV tachycardias associated with WPW syndrome as it increases conduction rate in accessory bundle
how to use?	• see p. 87

TREATMENT PLAN

note:
- a precise diagnosis is necessary before definitive treatment (ECG tracing essential)
- wide range of causes and of significance

general measures
- consider possible provoking factors such as smoking, alcohol, coffee, drugs, thyrotoxicosis and anxiety
- treatment primary cause

supraventricular tachycardia

for attack
- attempt unilateral carotid sinus pressure
- verapamil 5–10 mg i.v. over 2 min (NOT if patient is on beta-blockers)
- repeat 5 mg after 5 min if not controlled

D.C. shock if fails to respond

for prevention
- verapamil (by mouth) 120–360 mg daily, *or*
- atenolol 50–100 mg daily

atrial extrasystoles
- reassurance and explanation usually all that is required
- verapamil 120–360 mg daily, *or*
- atenolol 50–100 mg daily

atrial flutter
- digoxin as for cardiac failure (see Chapter 8) usually controls ventricular rate

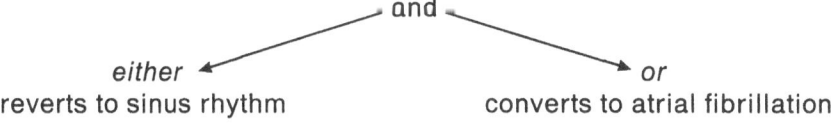

either	and	*or*
reverts to sinus rhythm		converts to atrial fibrillation

atrial fibrillation
- digoxin as for cardiac failure (see Chapter 8)
- *if urgent* (rarely and patient should be in hospital) digoxin 250 μg i.v. slowly and repeat in 2 h
- consider cardioversion
- anticoagulate in mitral stenosis

ventricular ectopics
- reassurance and explanation may be all that is necessary
- URGENT (multiple post-infarction)
  lignocaine 50–100 mg in i.v. bolus followed by infusion
- *non-urgent and for prevention*
  disopyramide – initially 100 mg three times daily

ventricular tachycardia
- usually serious – ADMIT urgently to hospital
- *attack*
  lignocaine 50–100 mg in i.v. bolus followed by infusion
  if no response – DC shock
- *prevention*
  disopyramide 100 mg three times daily, *or*
  amiodarone 600 mg daily for 1 week and then reduce to minimal
    effective dose

10 MIGRAINE

WHAT IS IT?

'Migraine' is a label for an imprecise syndrome of:

- episodic paroxysmal headaches
- headache may be unilateral but localization may be difficult
- nausea/vomiting
- prodromal aura – usually visual
- associated symptoms as yawning, mood changes, fluid retention followed by diuresis
- sometimes transient motor and/or sensory neurological disturbances
- migraine makes up about one-fifth of all headaches

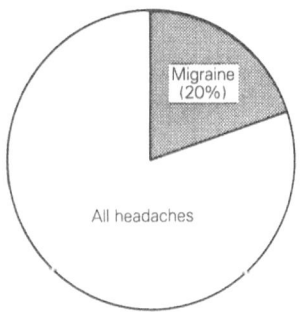

Migraine (20%)

All headaches

A clinical classification

Common migraine	=	mainly headache
Classical migraine	=	headache + nausea and vomiting
Complete migraine	=	aura + headache + nausea and vomiting
Migrainous neuralgia	=	cluster headaches with red eye and nasal symptoms
Complicated migraine	=	as above + transient hemiplegia, ophthalmoplegia or sensory symptoms

---

pathophysiology

- probably combination sequence of cerebral vasoconstriction followed by vasodilation

> - intracranial vasoconstriction → aura
> - extracranial dilation → headache, nausea and vomit

- underlying **migraine diathesis** in which triggers may produce attack through release of serotonin, kinin and catecholamines
- triggers may be:
  physical exhaustion
  mental stress
  foods as cheese, chocolate, alcohol, red wine, cured meats
  hormonal change (menstrual, contraceptive pill)

WHO GETS IT WHEN?

- women > men by 2 : 1
- social class 1 > 5
- 20% of population suffer from migraine
- **annual prevalence** in a general practice of 2500

Person ever suffering attacks	500
Persons consulting over 10 years	250
Annual prevalence of patients consulting	50
(Referred to hospital	1)
(Migrainous neuralgia	1–2)
(Complicated migraine	1 every 5 years)

- **onset** can be at any age but most often at 20–40 years

- **annual age prevalence**
  shows high frequency in women
  at 20–50 years

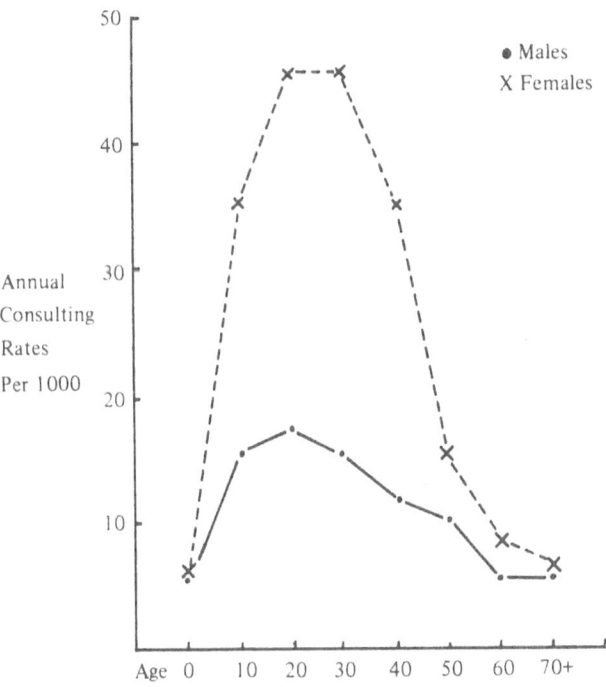

WHAT HAPPENS?

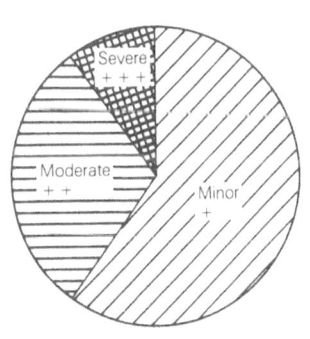

- tho natural history is for migraine attacks
  to cease spontaneously after a 'period of
  activity' of 10–20 years
- during **period of activity**
  in 10% of migraine it is severe
  in 30% of migraine it is moderate
  in 60% of migraine it is minor

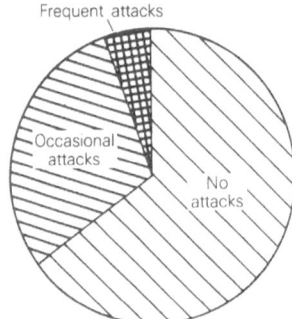

Frequent attacks

Occasional attacks

No attacks

- **assessment after 20 years from onset**
  in 65% attacks have ceased
  in 30% attacks occasional (1–2 per year)
  in 5% attacks frequent (at least every 3
     months)

MIGRAINE: A RECAP

- frequent condition (F > M)

- uncertain causes but with
  triggers in some individuals

- variety of clinical features and
  types

- most attacks cease
  spontaneously after 10–20 years

- during period of activity attacks
  may be disabling

WHAT TREATMENT?

objectives

- to relieve symptoms
  (i.e. headache and nausea)
  in acute attacks and long term

- to prevent attacks by
  self-help measures
  medication

- to correct very rare causes such
  as intracranial aneurysms or AV
  malformations

DRUGS FOR THE ACUTE ATTACK

SIMPLE ANALGESICS

what are they and how do they work?
- aspirin and paracetamol
- act as analgesics but also suppress prostaglandin synthesis, which may be important

effects

benefits
- adequate relief of headaches in 70% of patients

risks
- aspirin (see p. 9)
- paracetamol
  rashes and blood dyscrasias are rare
  overdose may cause hepatic and renal failure

which to use?
- do NOT use aspirin in persons with peptic ulcers, dyspepsias and who are on anticoagulants

how to use?
- take as early as possible at onset of attack
- most effective if combined with rest in a darkened room
- aspirin 300–900 mg every 4–6 h
- paracetamol 1 g every 4–6 h
- may be combined with metoclopramide

ANTI-EMETICS

what are they and how do they work?
- metoclopramide is most useful in combination with analgesic
- centrally acting anti-emetic may be related to dopamine blocking action
- increases gastric tone and shortens gastric emptying time

effects

benefits

- reduces vomiting in attack by speeding gastric emptying – hastens actions of analgesics

risks

- extrapyramidal symptoms (more often in young)
- facial spasm, oculogyric crises and unusual head movements
- cease on stopping drug and controlled by diazepam

how to use?

- take 10 min **before** analgesic
- **dose** adult: 10 mg tablet by mouth
  child: 2–5 years 2.0 mg
  6–14 years 2.5–5 mg
- **note**: combined analgesic and metoclopramide tablets available but no great advantages over giving drugs separately

ERGOTAMINE

what is it and how does it work?

- a vasoconstrictor that relieves headaches due to vasodilation
- combination with caffeine which may aid absorption

effects

benefits

- in one-third of attacks relieves headaches that do not respond to analgesics

risks

- **are appreciable and careful control of dosage is essential**
- **do NOT use** in pregnancy, lactation, renal and liver disease and in ischaemic heart disease

- **use with care** in peripheral vascular disease, which may be aggravated
- excessive dosing can cause intense vasoconstriction and gangrene
- nausea, vomiting and headaches both with too much drug or on withdrawal

what available and which to use?

- Cafergot: ergotamine 1 mg + caffeine per tablet
- Migril: ergotamine 2 mg + caffeine + cyclizine (anti-emetic) per tablet
- Cafergot suppository contains 2 mg of ergotamine
- Medihaler-ergotamine: 360 μg per puff
- **note**: oral preparations are best but there are different strengths per tablet

how to use?

- at onset of attack: 1–2 mg of ergotamine and repeat 1 mg every half hour if necessary to a daily maximum of 6 mg or 10 mg per week
- emphasize to patient that this regime is only for treatment of attack and not for regular long-term medication

SEDATIVES

- some migraine victims find a good sleep helps to relieve an attack
- a benzodiazepine (diazepam 5 mg) at onset of attack and if opportunity for sleep available

DRUGS FOR PREVENTION OF ATTACKS

β-ADRENERGIC BLOCKERS (see Chapter 6)

- mode of action in migraine is uncertain but may prevent vasodilation and tension

effects

benefits
- some prevention achieved in 50%

risks
- (see Chapter 6)

what to use and how?
- propranolol and atenolol are both effective – dose adjustment easier with atenolol
- atenolol 50–100 mg once daily
- propranolol 20 mg three times daily increased to 80 mg three times daily if necessary

PIZOTIFEN

what is it and how does it work?
- 5-hydroxytryptamine blocker
- related to tricyclic antidepressants
- probably alters vascular reactivity

effects

benefits
- used prophylactively is effective in preventing attacks

risks
- some anticholinergic action, so do NOT use in glaucoma and in prostatism
- causes sedation, increased appetite and weight gain

how to give?
- start with 500 μg three times daily or 1.5 mg as single night dose
- maximum daily dose 3 mg

CLONIDINE

what is it and how does it work?
- reduces reactivity of blood vessels
- in higher doses used as anti-hypertensive

effects

benefits

- reduces attacks in 70% of patients with classical migraine

risks

- may exacerbate or precipitate depression, dry mouth, sedation, dizziness, nausea
- do NOT combine with other anti-hypertensives

how to use?

- 50 μg twice daily and increase to 75 μg twice daily if necessary (in this dosage rebound hypertension is avoided)

SEDATIVES AND ANTIDEPRESSANTS

- **sedatives** are often used but any benefit is short lived with a risk of dependence
- **antidepressants** are not a treatment for migraine but may be useful for associated depression

TREATMENT PLAN

note:
- only 1 in 5 of all headaches are 'migraines' that may be expected to respond to specific therapies
- treatment is based on hypothesis of sensitive individuals reacting to certain trigger factors by sequence of vasoconstriction and then vasodilatation of cranial arteries
- in great majority 'migraine' is a temporary and self-limiting disorder

general measures
- avoid known predisposing factors or situations
- self-treat with simple effective measures at first symptoms of an attack

acute attack (general advice)
- commence treatment early during attack
- rest and sleep, if possible, in a darkened room
- short-acting benzodiazepine (temazepam 10 mg) may help to induce sleep – but care should be taken to avoid dependence with frequent attacks

mild-moderate attack
- aspirin 300–600 mg four to six hourly, *or*
- paracetamol 500 mg – 1 g four to six hourly
- analgesics may be combined with metaclopramide 10 mg to prevent nausea and vomiting
- co-codamol (paracetamol and codeine) two tablets six hourly may be more effective for some
- *note:* 'Migraleve' a combination of paracetamol, codeine, an anti-emetic and laxative can be used but is very similar to co-codamol plus metaclopramide

severe attack

ergotamine
- Cafergot: two tablets initially and then if not controlled one tablet every 30 min (maximum of six tablets in 24 h or ten per week)

- Cafergot suppositories: if vomiting present insert one and repeat in 2 h if no relief (maximum of three per day or five per week), *or*
- Migril tablets

prevention

- avoid known triggers (which may contain tyramine) such as:
  some cheeses
  some wines
  chocolates
  citrus fruits
- avoid situations which may trigger attacks:
  relaxation (at weekend)
  tension
  hunger
  menstruation
  exposure to sun (sun bathing)
- drugs which may predispose to attacks:
  the contraceptive pill – which should be given up if troublesome
  vasodilators (see Chapter 6)
- medication for prevention:
  (if more than two attacks per month)
  atenolol 50 mg daily (see p. 111)
  pizotifen 1.5 mg at night (see p. 112)
  clonidine 50–75 μg twice daily

outlook

- treatment plan is effective in about 60% of patients
- regime should be used for up to 6 months and then gradually tapored off
- occasionally antidepressant such as:
  amitriptyline 50 mg at night
  may be effective if depression is present

11 ASTHMA

WHAT IS IT?

- basic feature is a reversible partial occlusion of bronchi and bronchioles
- many possible 'triggers' that act on a hyper-responsive respiratory tract in 10% of whole population

clinical types

extrinsic (atopic) asthma

- children/teenagers
- eczema and hay fever in patient or family
- allergic-antigenic responses to dust, dust mites, pollen, grass, animal hair, drugs, foods
- IgE associated
- respond to mast-cell stabilisers
- good prognosis

intrinsic (non-atopic) asthma

- usually adult onset
- allergic-antigenic responses unusual
- IgE normal
- prognosis uncertain

others

- exercise induced
- occupational
- other diseases as chronic bronchitis

pathophysiology

- the essential feature of asthma is bronchial hyperactivity

- obstruction of airways due to bronchial oedema, increased secretion of mucus and constriction
- many factors may trigger this response but it is believed a number of mediators liberated from mast cells may play a central role in the asthmatic attack

WHO GETS IT WHEN?

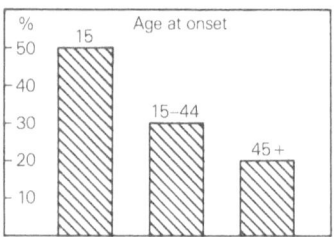

- half start asthma in childhood (0–14)
- one third at 15–44
- one quarter after 45

- *annual prevalence* in general practice of 2500

New cases	2–3
Attacks	50 (in 35 persons)
Asthmatics – with present or past history	250
Death from asthma	1 in 15 years

- age prevalence of attacks

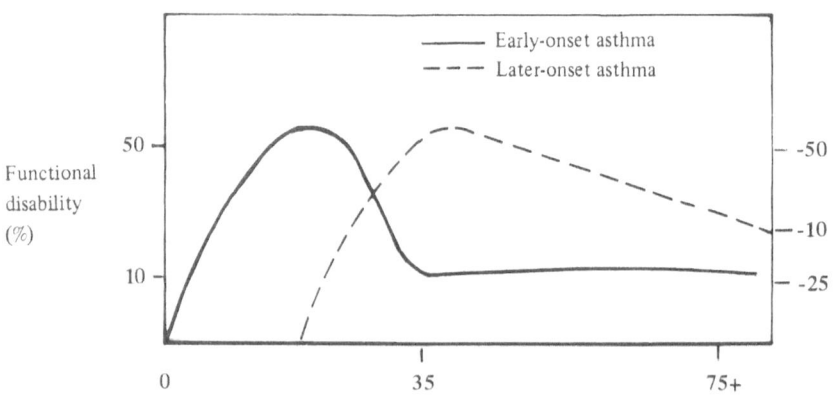

9 CARDIAC ARRHYTHMIA⁣

dia

WHAT ARE THEY?

- any disturbance of the hear
  cardiac arrhythmia
- may range from symptoms c
  sudden death
- may have cardiac or non-sp
- **cardiac**
  ischaemic heart disease
  cardiomyopathy
  mitral stenosis
  high blood presssure
  mitral valve prolapse
  Wolff–Parkinson–White syn

si

ve

- **non-cardiac**
  anxiety
  coffee, alcohol
  thyroid disease
  drugs
  smoking
  carcinoma of bronchus

ve

- **classification** (rate)
  tachycardias (>100 beats/m
  bradycardias (<60 beats/mi

s
a

site of origin

- **sinus**
  tachycardia
  bradycardia

a

- **supraventricular**
  atria: flutter
          fibrillation
  AV node: ectopics
            tachycardia

WHAT HAPPENS?

- generally a good prognosis – in many asthmatics attacks cease naturally
- differences of outcome in early and late onset asthma

early onset

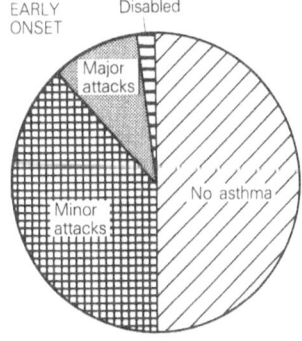

- in 50% attacks cease
- in 35% attacks are minor/infrequent
- in 12% they are major/frequent
- 3% respiratory invalids

late onset

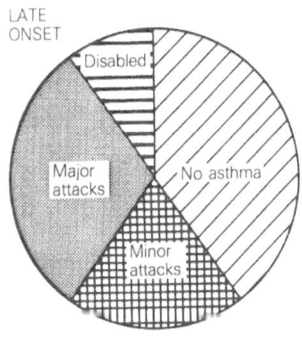

- in 40% attacks cease
- in 20% attacks are mild/infrequent
- in 30% they are major/frequent
- 10% respiratory invalids

ASTHMA: A RECAP

- frequent (10% of population)
- affects individuals with hyper-responsive respiratory tracts
- differences in extrinsic-early onset (atopic) and intrinsic-late onset (non-atopic) types
- generally good prognosis with 40–50% ceasing attacks naturally and less than 10% becoming respiratory invalids

---

WHAT TREATMENT?

objectives
- to control acute attacks
- to avoid and prevent attacks
- to maintain normal life and function
- to plan for natural remission
- to prevent death

DRUGS

SELECTIVE β_2-RECEPTOR STIMULANTS

what are they and how do they work?
- competitive stimulation of β_2-receptors producing bronchodilatation
- in high dosage some β_1-stimulation with tachycardia

effects

benefits
- safe and effective bronchodilators in asthma and in bronchospasm in chronic bronchitis
- used to **relieve** asthmatic attacks and also to prevent attacks either before provocation (e.g. exercise) or on a regular basis

risks
- used correctly by inhalation they are very safe
- true tolerance is unlikely to develop but very severe asthma may not respond

adverse effects
- due to β_1-stimulation:
  tachycardia
  tremor
  nervousness
  insomnia
  muscle cramps
- these can be reduced by lowering dose

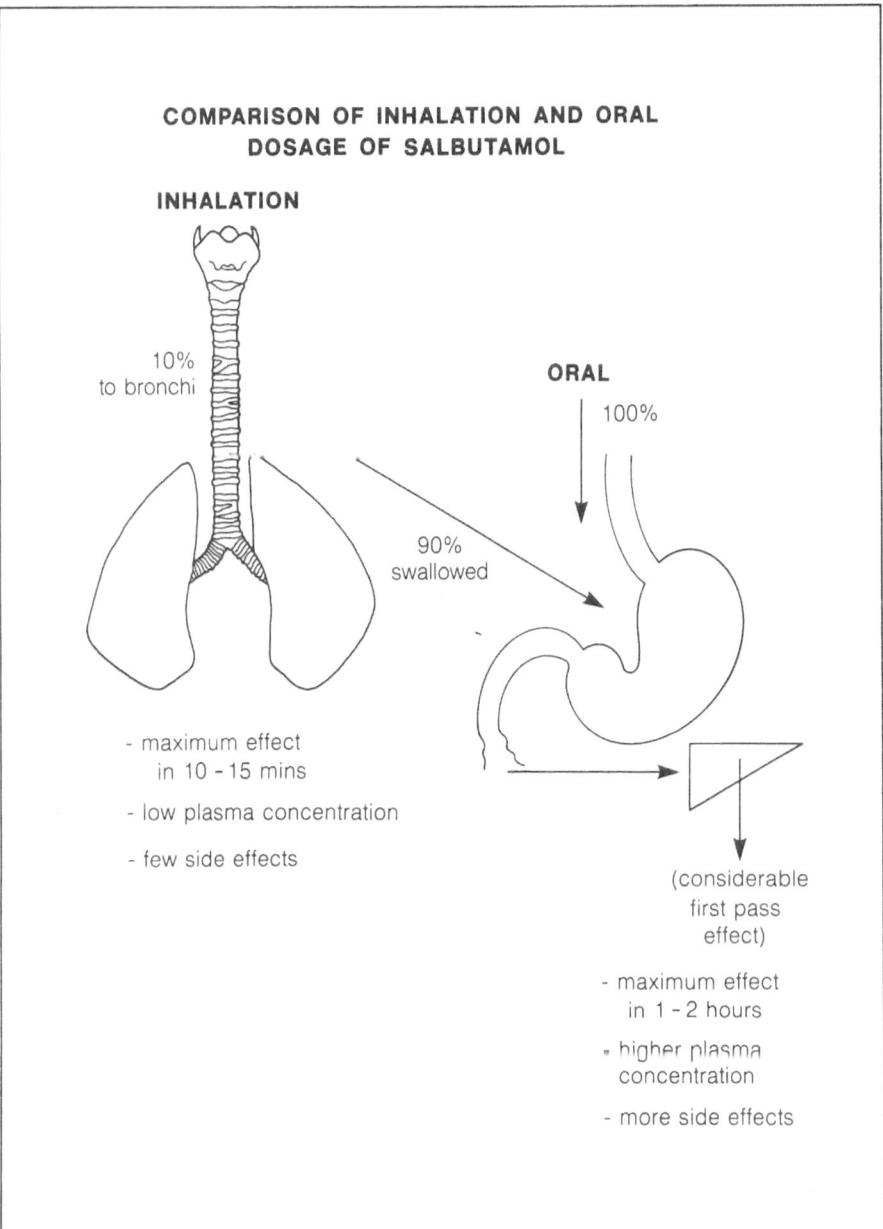

COMPARISON OF INHALATION AND ORAL DOSAGE OF SALBUTAMOL

INHALATION

10%
to bronchi

ORAL

100%

90%
swallowed

- maximum effect
  in 10 - 15 mins

- low plasma concentration

- few side effects

(considerable
first pass
effect)

- maximum effect
  in 1 - 2 hours

- higher plasma
  concentration

- more side effects

interactions

- benefits are reduced by beta-blockers
- **note**: do NOT use in thyrotoxicosis or severe hypertension

what available?

- many preparations – all are very similar

Drug	Dose of aerosol for regular use (daily)
Fenoterol	200–400 μg : 3 to 4 times
Orciprenaline[a]	750–1500 μg : 4 to 6 times
Pirbuterol	200–400 μg : 3 to 4 times
Reproterol	0.5–1.0 mg : 3 times
Rimiterol	200–600 μg : 3 to 4 times
Salbutamol	200 μg : 3 to 4 times
Terbutaline	250–500 μg : 3 to 4 times

[a] orciprenaline has a more marked β_1-(cardiac) effect

which to use?

- salbutamol is most popular
- pirbuterol is very similar
- terbutaline is available with a spacer
- fenoterol is longer acting

how to use?

- inhalation is safest and most effective route
- only 10–15% of inhaled dose reaches the bronchi
- routes for salbutamol are shown as an example

salbutamol: aerosol inhaler

- **for adults**
  two puffs (200 μg) three to four times daily

- **for children**
  one puff (100 μg) three to four times daily

- **children under ten**
  aerosol difficult to use

salbutamol: rotahaler

- **for adult**
  400 μg three to four times daily

- **for children**
  200 μg three to four times daily

- beneficial effects last for 2–4 h – in some circumstances three hourly inhalations may be justifiable for a short while

salbutamol: nebulizer

- more effective delivery system than aerosol

- 1 ml of respiratory solution (5.0 mg salbutamol) diluted to 4 ml with sterile saline and inhaled through nebulizer

- airflow of 6–8 l/min for optimum particle size

- repeat four to six hourly if necessary

- *note*: there are risks in home use of nebulizers, asthmatics may delay call for further help in severe attacks requiring hospital care

spacer

- note: spacer for terbutaline: where difficulty with aerosols or rotacaps a **spacer** acts as a reservoir between aerosol and mouthpiece

salbutamol: oral

- more side effects likely with less therapeutic benefits

- **for adult**
  8 mg in a slow release preparation (Spandets) once or twice daily and 8–16 mg at night for nocturnal attacks

- **for children**
  sugar-free syrup is available (2 mg per 5 ml)

2–6 years	1–2 mg
6–12 years	2 mg
over 12	2–4 mg

salbutamol: by injection

- **for adult**
- intramuscular 500 μg four hourly
- intravenous 250 μg in 5 ml, administer slowly
  indication: for severe attack when inhalation is ineffective – patient should be in hospital on a cardiac monitor

METHYLXANTHINES

what are they and how do they work?

- theophylline and aminophylline
- relax bronchial muscles
- weak diuretic and cerebral stimulants

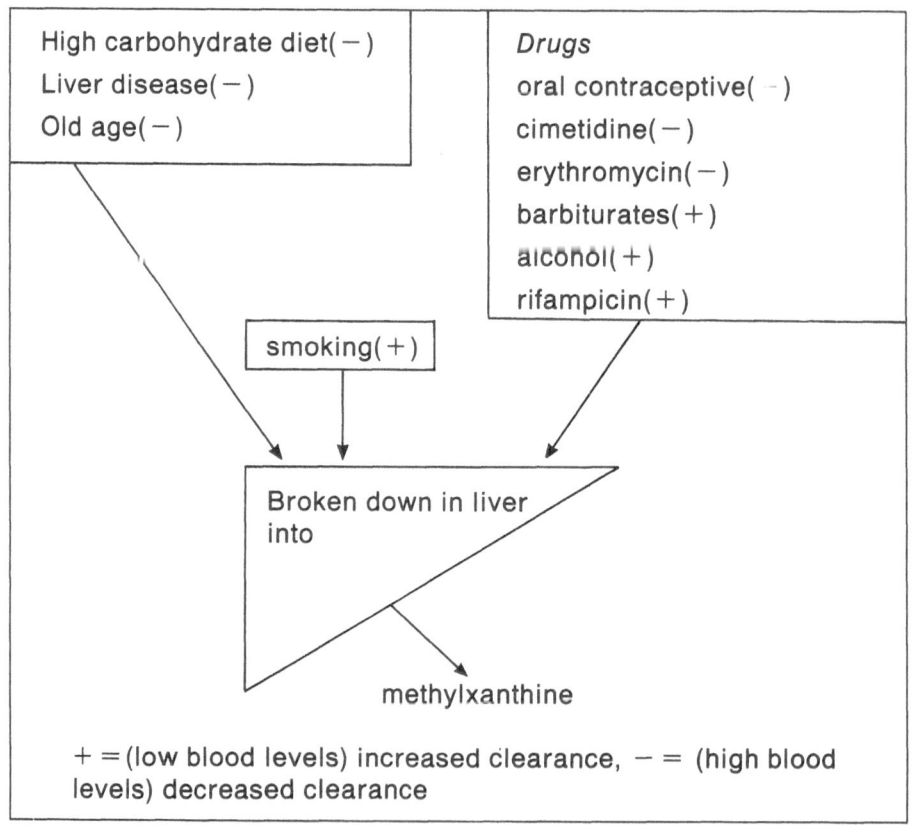

High carbohydrate diet(−)
Liver disease(−)
Old age(−)

Drugs
oral contraceptive(−)
cimetidine(−)
erythromycin(−)
barbiturates(+)
alcohol(+)
rifampicin(+)

smoking(+)

Broken down in liver into

methylxanthine

+ = (low blood levels) increased clearance, − = (high blood levels) decreased clearance

- **metabolism in liver** is modified by age, smoking, diet, liver disease and concurrent drugs
- therefore variable half life (3–10 h) and duration of action and variable plasma levels (therapeutic range 10–20 mg/l)
- because of low therapeutic index there is danger of toxicity

effects

benefits

- used **orally** to prevent asthma attacks, particularly at night
- duration of action 4–8 h, or longer with slow-release preparations
- can be used **intravenously** if unresponsive to other measures for severe asthma attack
- use in chronic bronchitics is controversial and requires careful monitoring

risks

- are dose related
- nausea and vomiting
- cardiac arrhythmias
- sleep interference
- fits
- **note**: particular danger of intravenous aminophylline in patient already on oral methylxanthines

what available?

- slow-release (SR) tablets are less nauseating
- many preparations, e.g.
    aminophylline SR
    theophylline SR
    theophylline liquid
- *also* aminophylline injection

| **which to use?** | • no specially preferred preparation |

| **how to use?** | • aminophylline SR 225 mg twice daily (or only at night and this may be doubled after a week) |

• **for children**
4–8   years 100 mg twice daily
8–13 years 100–200 mg twice daily

• theophylline SR 400 mg once daily for adults (may be doubled after a week)

• **note**: ideally to obtain optimum results and avoid toxicity start with low dose and measure blood levels after 6 days and 4 h after the last dose – adjust dose to obtain levels of 10–20 mg/l. Check levels every 6 months.

• **note**: do NOT use orally in acute attack

intravenous

• only to be used in acute attacks

• if patient already on a methylxanthine then either try some other treatment or give half dose

• slow administration (over 10 min) 200–250 mg

• half dose for frail and olderly and those with liver disease

• continuous infusion – 250 mg over 6 h (according to weight) (check plasma levels after 24 h)

IPRATROPIUM BROMIDE

what is it and how does it work?

• anticholinergic agent acting predominantly on bronchial muscles with relaxation

• poorly absorbed orally and has to be inhaled

• acts in 30 min and effects last for 3–4 h

126

effects

benefits
- most effective in elderly asthmatics and bronchitics and in preventing bronchospasm

risks
- risks are unusual
- dry mouth
- unpleasant taste
- constipation
- urinary retention

how to use?
- aerosol inhaler 18–36 μg (one or two puffs) three to four times daily
- best results if inhaled 10 min after inhaling salbutamol (or similar drug)

SODIUM CROMOGLYCATE

what is it and how does it work?
- an asthma prophylactic in allergic asthma, particularly children
- stabilizes mast cell membranes and prevents release of mediators of bronchospasm

effects

benefits
- with regular use prevents attacks including exercise asthma
- although most effective in extrinsic (allergy) asthma may help in late-onset asthma

risks
- few
- inhaled powder may be irritant and cause bronchospasm

what available?	• sodium cromoglycate insufflation cartridges (spincaps) containing 20 mg
	• sodium cromoglycate aerosol inhalers 1.0 and 5.0 mg per puff (also available with isoprenaline)
how to use?	• insufflation cartridge 20 mg: three to four times daily
	• aerosol 2–10 mg: four to six times daily
	• to prevent exercise asthma use half hour before the exercise
	• **for children** 20 mg: three to four times daily by insufflator

NEDOCROMIL

what is it and how does it work?	• an asthma prophylactic
	• stabilizes cell membranes of many inflammatory cells
	• also blocks mediator release and has effects on the neural pathways of inflammation

effects

benefits	• prevents attacks with regular use
	• if given with steroids it may allow a reduction in steroid dosage or even complete withdrawal
	• effective in both intrinsic and extrinsic asthma
risks	• few risks
	• may produce an unpleasant taste in the mouth
what available?	• metered dose aerosol (2 mg per puff)

how to use?	• two puffs twice daily increasing if necessary to two puffs four times a day

CORTICOSTEROIDS

what are they and how do they work?	• relieve by reducing bronchial oedema and hypersecretion
	• may block allergic responses and reduce bronchospasm

effects

benefits	• very effective in *acute asthma* but act only after 3–5 h
	• *prevent* asthma when taken regularly
	• may *relieve* bronchospasm in a few chronic bronchitics
risks	• systemic administration: can lead to steroid effects if taken long term
	• inhalation can cause oral candidiasis

what available and which to use?	• oral tablets – prednisolone or prednisone
	• inhalation beclomethasone dipropionate aerosol: 50 μg/puff rotacap: 100–200 μg per capsule high dose aerosol: 250 μg per puff

how to use?

severe acute attack	• hydrocortisone hemisuccinate 200 mg i.v. (children 100 mg i.v.) every 4 h
preventive	• aerosol inhaler 200 μg (four puffs) twice daily – equivalent to 8 mg oral prednisolone

- **for children**
  100 μg twice daily
- by rotacap: 100 μg two to four times daily
- may be more effective if preceded by β_2-agonist

oral steroids for deteriorating asthma
- prednisolone 30 mg on first 2 days and reduce and phase out over 8 days

for resistant asthma
- endeavour to keep below 8 mg daily (risk of systemic side effects with prolonged higher dosage)
- give as single early morning dose to minimize adrenal suppression

TREATMENT PLAN

note:
- different types of asthma at different ages with differing natural histories and prognoses
- *best* prognosis in extrinsic types and in young
- *worse* in intrinsic types and in elderly

general measures
- long-term care and supervision necessary so an 'asthma' register is useful
- asthma is a disorder requiring self-understanding and self-care and an effective use of the various drugs
- importance of subjective measures of respiratory function – therefore instruct in use of own peak flow meters
- make sure diagnosis is correct and exclude other causes (by investigation) and try and discover avoidable causal triggers (pets, pollen, other allergens)
- ensure patients and family know the difference between *preventive* and *therapeutic* drugs
- ensure patients and family use inhalers and nebulizers effectively

acute severe attack
- life threatening with appreciable mortality therefore ADMIT urgently to hospital unit with appropriate resources

high risk features
- too breathless to speak
- pulse rate > 130 per min
- cyanosis
- silent chest
- pulsus paradoxus

emergency treatment at home
- oxygen if available (2 l/mln)
- hydrocortisone succinate 200 mg i.v. four hourly followed by oral prednisolone 40 mg on first day and reducing

- salbutamol by nebulizer (if available): 5 mg salbutamol in 4 ml saline

if this fails

- salbutamol 500 μg i.m. *or*
- aminophylline 250 mg i.v. (for adult) over 5 min – provided patient is NOT on methylxanthine

chronic asthma in adults

- stress need for regular monitoring of peak respiratory flow rates
- *intermittent attacks*: β_2-antagonist inhalers as required:
    aerosol
    rotahaler
    home nebulizer
- nebulizers are efficient, but require careful monitoring and are not necessary for most asthmatics at home – also failure to respond to nebulized β_2-antagonists means condition is dangerous
- daily peak flow monitoring is essential with nebulizers to spot deterioration
- *escalating asthma*
    short course of oral steroids
    may need long-term with dose < 8 mg daily
- *noctural asthma*
    slow release oral β_2-antagonists
    slow release oral methylxanthine
- *exercise asthma*
    β_2-antagonist inhaler *or*
    sodium cromoglycate inhaler
    to be used before exercise
- *prevention*
    β_2-antagonist inhaler three to four times daily
    sodium cromoglycate inhaler three to four times daily
    oral methylxanthine
- *note*: *antibiotics* may be given if infection implicated but usually not helpful as infection is probably virus (antibiotics are no substitute for bronchodilators)

asthma in children
general

- usually extrinsic-atopic type but not all that wheezes is true asthma

severe attack

- treat as early as possible
- short course of oral steroids
- β_2-antagonist by nebulizer or rotahaler
- consider hospital admission

moderate–mild attack

- β_2-antagonist
  over 9 years: use aerosol
  3–9 years: use nebulizer or rotahaler
  under 3 years: use nebulizer
- if these routes not possible, then use oral preparations

preventive

- use preventive measures when
  asthma interfering with normal life routines
  frequent/severe attacks
  persistent airways obstruction
- sodium cromoglycate by inhalation – regular
- β_2-antagonist by mouth or inhalation – also helpful in exercise-induced attacks
- steroids by inhalation

(*note*: careful monitoring with peak flow meter is important and immediate use of short course of steroids for a deteriorating situation may prevent progression of attack)

asthma in elderly

note: response to bronchodilators is often poor

- β_2-antagonists by aerosol, nebulizer or rotahaler
- check that inhaler equipment is being used properly – lack of response may be due to faulty technique
- ipratropium may be more effective in this age group
- do not delay use of oral steroids if poor response to bronchodilators
- home supply of oxygen may be necessary

COMMON ACUTE INFECTIONS

WHAT ARE THEY?

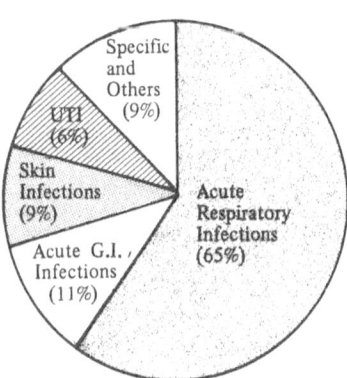

- **infections** are common and the most common acute infections are, in order of frequency, those affecting:

  - respiratory tract
  - gastrointestinal tract
  - skin
  - urinary tract
  - others, such as specific fevers, gynaecological infections, infectious mononucleosis, hepatitis, eye infections, tuberculosis, meningitis, etc.

- **in theory** it should be possible to allocate a specific organism as the cause of the infection

- **in practice** this is impossible because in many apparent infections no pathogen can be isolated even when intensive investigations are carried out

upper respiratory infections

- most are presumed to be caused by 'viruses' but few pathogens can be identified during attacks and few produce definitive clinical syndromes – exceptions are epidemic influenza and infectious mononucleosis

acute tonsillitis:

> - in about $\frac{1}{3}$ *Streptococcus pyogenes* is isolated
> - in $\frac{2}{3}$ no pathogens are detected

acute otitis media:

> - in $\frac{1}{3}$ *Haemophilus influenzae* can be isolated
> - in $\frac{1}{6}$ a pneumococcus or streptococcus
> - in $\frac{1}{2}$ no pathogens isolated

gastrointestinal infections

- in the great majority no specific pathogens are to be found

> - in $\frac{9}{10}$ no pathogens
> - in $\frac{1}{10}$ possibly pathogenic *E. coli*, dysentery, salmonella or *Giardia*

skin infections

- the situation is different:

> - in more than $\frac{9}{10}$ staphylococci or streptococci isolated
> - in $\frac{1}{10}$ other pathogens such as *Pseudomonas* spp.

urinary tract infections

> - in $\frac{1}{2}$ no pathogenic bacteria found
> - in $\frac{1}{3}$ *E. coli*
> - in $\frac{1}{6}$ various pathogens such as staphylococci, *Strep. faecalis*, *Proteus*, *Pseudomonas* spp., *Klebsiella*

who gets them when?

- almost one-half (46%) of the population visits their family doctor each year for treatment of infections

- persons consulting annually for infections in a population of 2500

Site	Numbers consulting
Respiratory tract	775
GI tract	125
Skin	110
Urinary tract	65
Others	75
Total	1150

- the **age prevalence rates** differ in the various infections

- **respiratory infections** are most prevalent in childhood and then become less frequent

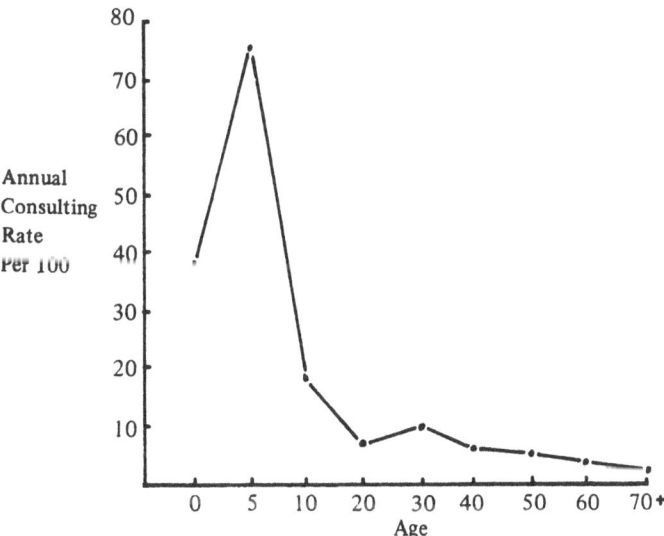

- **gastrointestinal infections** are most prevalent in childhood but remain frequent throughout life

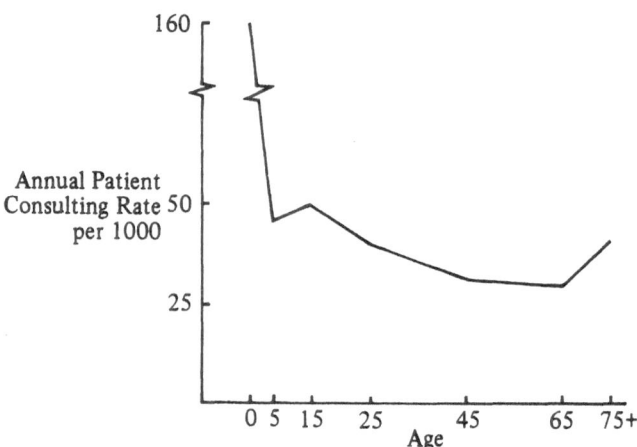

- **skin infections** are most prevalent in childhood

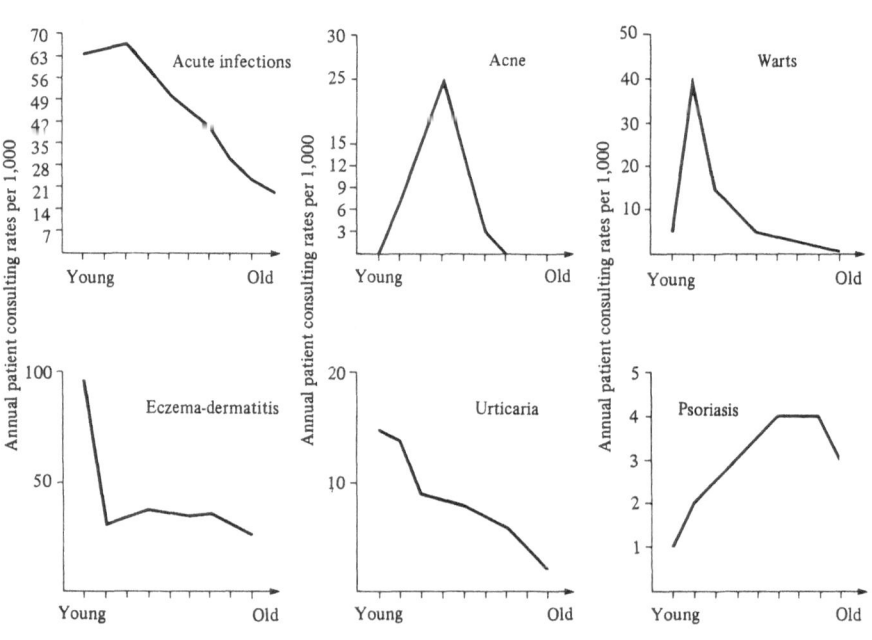

- urinary tract infections
  in females frequent in early and mid-adult life
  in males most prevalent in elderly men

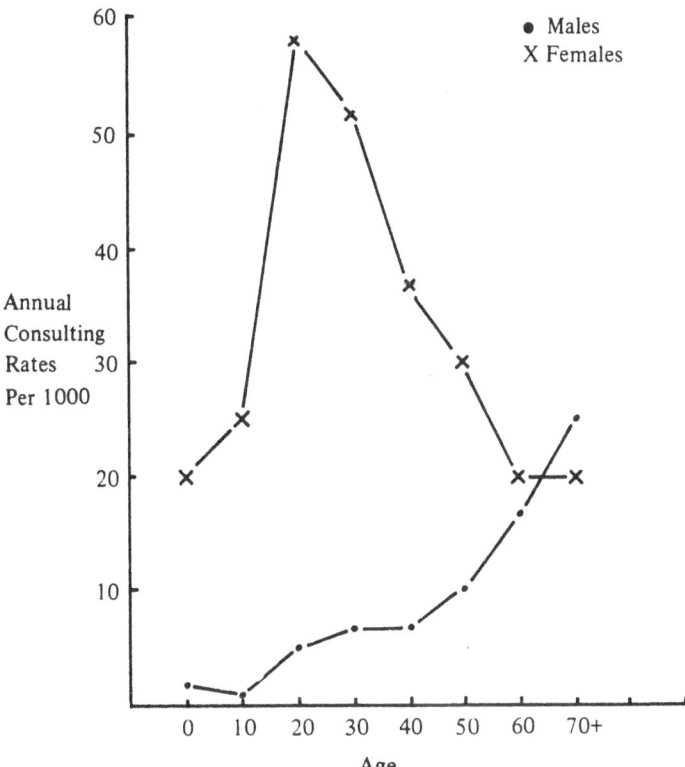

what happens?

- it must be stressed that normally the body's defences against infection are good and probably that almost all of the common acute infections would recover naturally

- it has also be to noted that the **virulence** of common organisms, such as streptococci, has changed and they are less dangerous in their effects than in the past

- it has also to be noted that in developed Western societies the **general health and resistance of the hosts**, the people, is greater than in the less developed societies
- it has also to be noted that there are now available powerful **antibiotics** against most pathogenic bacteria associated with the common infections
- common infections should, therefore, present fewer problems in management – but paradoxically they still raise questions

---

COMMON INFECTIONS: A RECAP
- one half of the population attend for treatment of infections each year
- the most frequent sites are:
    respiratory
    gastrointestinal
    skin
    urinary tract
- in many clinical infections no pathogen can be isolated
- in general infections are less virulent and dangerous than in the past

---

WHAT TREATMENT?

---

objectives
- to control infection
- to promote resolution of infection
- to prevent complications
- to use antibiotics sensibly
- to avoid side-effects of treatment

PRINCIPLES

general measures

- accept that the healthy human body can control and overcome most common acute infections naturally

- accept that in clinical practice no pathogenic bacteria (sensitive to antibiotics) may be detected in many common infections

- local measures can assist natural processes, e.g. rest, pain relief

drugs

- antibiotics and chemotherapy are available for most common infections

- key decisions are when to use antibiotics, which antibiotic, how and for how long?

DRUGS: ANTIBIOTICS

note: doses are given under individual infections

THE PENICILLINS

what are they and how do they work?

- large group of antibiotics with common basic structure
- prevent the build up of the wall of bacteria
- several types with differing antibacterial spectra and uses

benzylpenicillin
procaine penicillin
phenoxymethylpenicillin
(Penicillin V)

effects

benefits

- effective in streptococcal infections (tonsillitis and erysipelas) *and*
- pneumococcal infections
- meningococcal meningitis
- gonococcal infections
- syphilis

risks

(see p. 143)

how to use?

benzylpenicillin
- ineffective orally and rapidly excreted
- twice daily i.m. injections (painful) are adequate for sensitive organisms, but more frequent dosage (or i.v. infusion) in serious infections
- more than 1.2 g (2 megaunits) is very painful i.m. and i.v. infusion is kinder

procaine penicillin
- slow release
- twice daily injections are adequate

phenoxymethylpenicillin
- oral, only suitable if organisms are sensitive and patient not vomiting
- poorly absorbed so must be given half hour before food

penicillinase resistant penicillins

flucloxacillin
- effective against penicillinase (β-lactamase) producing staphylococci and should be reserved for treating infections when this organism is likely cause
- otherwise similar antibacterial range but rather less effective than benzylpenicillin
- usually given orally but parenteral preparations available for severe infection

extended range penicillins

| ampicillin |
| amoxycillin |
| Augmentin |
| (amoxycillin and clavulanic acid) |

- wider antibacterial range than benzylpenicillin and effective against some gram-negative organisms (e.g. *E. coli* and *H. influenzae*)
- effective in:
  acute bronchitis
  most pneumonias (but NOT staphylococcal, mycoplasma and *Legionella*)
  acute otitis media

sinusitis
urinary tract infections
most biliary infections
prevention of bacterial endocarditis with
dental treatment

amoxycillin

- better absorbed but more expensive than ampicillin
- given orally, but by injection for serious infections

Augmentin

- effective against β-lactamase penicillinase producing organisms (e.g. some strains of *H. influenzae*) – clavulanic acid inactivates β-lactamase
- more likely to cause diarrhoea
- reserve for special circumstance

Magnapen

- mixture of ampicillin and flucloxacillin
- oral and by injection
- NOT for routine use but can be considered if causal organism in doubt

broad spectrum antipseudomonal penicillins

piperacillin
azlocillin
ticarallin
mezlocillin

- group of expensive penicillins with greater activity against Gram-negative organisms
- effective against *Pseudomonas aeruginosa*
- should be reserved for serious infections
- inactivated by penicillinase
- all must be given by injection or infusion

risks with all penicillins

- anaphylactic reactions in 1 : 5000 persons (with 10% mortality) – therefore *always* ask about previous sensitivities

- serum sickness or Stevens–Johnson syndrome in 2%
- specific maculopapular rash usually late in treatment, or after stopping, with ampicillin or amoxycillin – especially in infectious mononucleosis or lymphomas
- diarrhoea – frequent after oral ampicillin or amoxycillin
- thrush – vaginal after ampicillin or amoxycillin
- fits – in patients with renal failure, due to accumulation
- oral contraceptive activity may be reduced occasionally
- local applications – hypersensitivity reactions
- haemolytic anaemias – rare

CEPHALOSPORINS

what are they and how do they work?
- similar to penicillins
- many available, some with wide antibacterial range
- not widely used because cheaper and equally good substitutes available and most have to be injected·
- two useful ones are **cefadroxil** and **cefuroxime**

cefadroxil
- effective in:
  urinary tract infections (*E. coli*)
  respiratory infections (*H. influenzae*, pneumococci)
  skin infections (streptococci and staphylococci including some penicillinase producing strains)
- given orally: 500 mg–1 g twice daily but less in renal failure

COMMON ACUTE INFECTIONS

cefuroxime	• effective in wide range of infections (*E. coli, H. influenzae, N. gonococci* and staphylococci – (including penicillinase-producing strains)
	• reserved for serious infections, particularly if organism not isolated
	• usually given in combination with other antibiotic
	• effective in common types of meningitis
	• 750 mg by injection eight hourly (painful)

Activities of some other cephalosporins

	S. aureus	*Penicillinase stability*	H. influenzae	E. coli	Pseudo-monas	*Anaerobes*
Cephazolin	+ +	+	+	+ +	−	−
Cephamandole	+ +	+	+ +	+ +	−	−
Cefoxitin	+	+ +	+	+ +	−	−
Cefotaxime	+	+ +	+ +	+ +	+	+
Latamoxef	+	+ +	+ +	+	+	+ +
Ceftazidime	+	+ +	+ +	+ +	+ +	+

+ + bacteria sensitive; + some strains sensitive; − bacteria insensitive
Note: These have a place in special situations but should not be used as first line antibiotics

risks	• similar to penicillins
	rashes
	nausea
	diarrhoea
	• **note**: 10% of penicillin-sensitive persons are also sensitive to cephalosporins – do NOT use where history of penicillin reactions

ERYTHROMYCIN

what is it and how does it work?
• one of the macrolides group of antibiotics
• inhibits bacterial protein synthesis

	• similar antibacterial spectrum to benzylpenicillin
	• useful in penicillin-sensitive patients
effective in:	• respiratory infections, including staphylococcal pneumonia
	• *Mycoplasma pneumoniae* and Legionnaire's disease
	• prevention of bacterial endocarditis with dental treatment
	• given orally with food
adverse effects	• nausea
	• potentiates action of theophylline
	• rarely jaundice

TETRACYCLINES

what are they and how do they work?	• act by inhibiting bacterial protein synthesis
	• wide antibacterial range
	• bacterial resistance common
effective in:	• exacerbations of chronic bronchitis
	• non-specific urethritis
	• *Mycoplasma pneumoniae*
	• acne (reason not known)
	• given orally before meals four times a day
adverse effects	• exacerbate renal failure
	• tooth staining in children and in foetus (when given to mother) (do NOT use in pregnancy or for children <8 years)
	• nausea

- superinfection by *Candida*
- diarrhoea
- raised intracranial pressure in infants (rare)

GENTAMICIN

what is it and how does it work?
- an aminoglycoside
- inhibits bacterial protein synthesis

effective in:
- Gram-negative infections, e.g. *Proteus*, *Pseudomonas* and *E. coli*, and *Klebsiella* spp.
- staphylococcal infections
- *not* streptococci or pneumococci except when combined with penicillin in *Streptococcus viridans* endocarditis
- reserved for serious infections when simpler antibiotics are ineffective

- given by injection i.m. or i.v.
- reduced dose with renal impairment – remember renal function may decline during an infection
- the initial dose is 80 mg for adults more than 60 kg in weight or 60 mg where less than 60 kg in weight or elderly. Initial dose does not depend on renal function
- in emergency can be given before admission to hospital
- subsequent doses depend on elimination rate
- narrow therapeutic range, so blood levels need to be monitored for best peak and trough levels, i.e. $\frac{1}{2}$ h after injection and before injection (frequency depends on clinical situation but at least twice weekly)

adverse effects	• ototoxic – related to length of exposure and blood levels
	• nephrotoxic – especially when combined with diuretics and some cephalosporins
	• rashes
	• potentiates effects of curare-like muscle relaxants

SODIUM FUSIDATE

what is it and how does it work?	• interferes with bacterial protein synthesis
	• effective in staphylococcal infections, including penicillinase-producing organisms
	• given orally, usually combined with another anti-staphylococcal drug such as erythromycin or flucloxacillin, to prevent development of resistance
	• use only in serious infections
adverse effects	• nausea
	• rashes
	• jaundice in high dose systemic administration – clears on stopping drug

TRIMETHOPRIM
CO-TRIMOXAZOLE (trimethoprim 80 mg and sulphamethoxazole 400 mg per tablet)

what are they and how do they work?	• interfere with bacterial folate production
	• co-trimoxazole combines two antibacterials with objective of more effectiveness and prevention of resistant strains developing

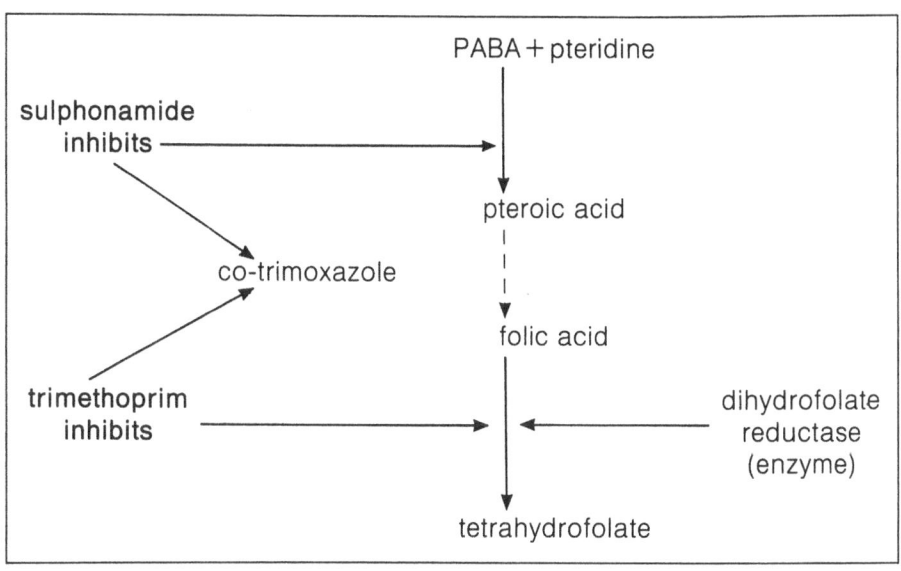

Sites of action of sulphonamide and trimethroprim

effective in:

- **both** in urinary infections (*E. coli*)
- co-trimoxazole in
  respiratory infections
  prostatitis
  enteric fever
  pneumocystis (high dosage)
- given orally (lower doses if creatinine clearance is less than 25 ml/min)

adverse effects

- nausea
- rashes
- Stevens–Johnson syndrome
- do NOT use in pregnancy (trimethoprim in first trimester; co-trimoxazole in 1 and 3 trimesters) or in neonates
- **note**: adverse effects are common with co-trimoxazole, trimethoprim alone is to be preferred for urinary infections

TREATMENT PLAN FOR RESPIRATORY TRACT INFECTIONS WITH ANTIBIOTICS

pharyngitis and tonsillitis

- *note*: most throat infections are non-bacterial and should be treated symptomatically

- *for adults*
  aspirin 300–600 mg four to six hourly
  paracetamol 500 mg–1 g four to six hourly

- *for children*
  paracetamol (per dose)
  up to 1 year 60–120 mg
  1–5 years 120–250 mg
  6–12 years 250–500 mg
  Elixir (120 mg/5 ml) available

in likely or proven streptococcal infections

- *for adults*
  phenoxymethylpenicillin orally 250–500 mg six hourly, *or*
  benzylpenicillin 600 mg i.m. twice daily

- *for children*
  phenoxymethylpenicillin – dose given six hourly
  up to 1 year 62.5 mg
  1–5 years 125 mg
  6–12 years 250 mg
  (if child vomiting benzylpenicillin 20 mg/kg i.m. twice daily until vomiting ceases)

acute otitis media and sinusitis

- may be caused by streptococci and *H. influenzae* but in many cases no bacterial pathogens isolated

if antibiotics considered necessary

- *for adult*
  ampicillin 500 mg or amoxycillin 250 mg eight hourly
  erythromycin 500 mg six hourly (if penicillin sensitive)

- for *children*
  all doses to be given eight hourly
  - amoxycillin
    - 0–1 years 62.5 mg
    - 1–7 years 125 mg
    - 7+ years 250 mg
  (*note*: syrups 125 and 250 mg per 5 ml)
  - erythromycin (for penicillin sensitive)
    - 0–2 years 125 mg
    - 2–7 years 250 mg
    - 7+ years 500 mg
  (*note*: syrups 125 and 250 mg per 5 ml)
  all doses given six-hourly

acute bronchitis

note: probably often non-bacterial (viral?) and/or part of asthma syndrome

if antibiotics considered necessary

- for *adult*
  ampicillin 500 mg or amoxycillin 250 mg eight hourly
  erythromycin 500 mg six hourly
- for *children*
  (as for acute otitis media)

acute exacerbations of chronic bronchitis

- ampicillin 500 mg or amoxycillin 250 mg eight hourly *or* (if ineffective or penicillin-sensitive patient)
- co-trimoxazole two tablets twice daily for 5 days
- start treatment as soon as possible in attack
- with recurring attacks patient should be supplied with antibacterial drug and instructions to start whenever cough increases with purulent sputum

acute pneumonias

- causal organisms usually not determined in general practice, but sputum bacteriology and blood culture are checked in hospitals
- most likely organisms are pneumococci and *H. influenzae*, and staphylococci during epidemics of influenza
- treat the degree of illness rather than the signs

for children

- amoxycillin
- erythromycin (if penicillin sensitive)
  (as for acute otitis media)

for adult

- amoxycillin 500 mg by mouth eight hourly
- if *penicillin sensitive* then
  erythromycin 500 mg six hourly
- if likely to be staphylococcal then *add* flucloxacillin 500 mg six hourly
- treatment for at least 1 week, but if no response in 48 h, review the regime

in very ill adult patient – particularly in previously fit individual

- possible causes include pneumococci, *Legionella* and staphylococci (particularly during epidemics of influenza)
- therefore to cover these possibilities give:
  amoxycillin 500 mg six hourly
  (orally or i.v. if necessary) *and*
  erythromycin 500 mg six hourly
  (orally or i.v. if necessary)
- regime must be reviewed day by day in light of response and admission to hospital is likely:
  staphylococci will need addition of flucloxacillin 500 mg six hourly
  Legionella, the addition of rifampicin 600 mg daily for 3 days

TREATMENT PLAN FOR URINARY TRACT INFECTIONS

acute (uncomplicated) cystitis

- in one half no pathogenic organisms isolated
- in one third usually *E. coli* isolated
- preliminary culture is the ideal but not essential in uncomplicated attacks

for adult
- trimethoprim 200 mg 12 hourly with high fluid intake or
- co-trimoxazole two tablets 12 hourly or
- ampicillin/amoxycillin 250 mg eight hourly
- in pregnancy do NOT use:
  trimethoprim (first trimester) or co-trimoxazole (1 and 3 trimesters)
- three days treatment usually sufficient

for children
- ampicillin/amoxycillin
  (doses given eight hourly)
  0–1 years   62.5 mg
  1–7 years 125 mg
  7 + years 250 mg
- cefadroxil
  (doses given twice daily)
  0–1 years   12.5 mg/kg
  1–6 years 250 mg
  6 + years 500 mg
  (*note*: syrup with 125 and 250 mg per 5 ml)
- trimethoprim
  (doses given twice daily)
  6 weeks–5 months 4 mg/kg (about 25 mg)
  6 months–5 years 50 mg
  6 years–12 years 100 mg
  12 + years 200 mg
  (*note*: suspension with 50 mg per 5 ml)

acute pyelonephritis

- as above for seven days but in serious infections *add*:
- gentamicin (*adult*: 60–80 mg i.m. eight-hourly) but this must be controlled by blood levels

preventive

for adult

- trimethoprim 100 mg at night
- nitrofurantoin 100 mg at night with food but do NOT use in renal failure

for children

- trimethoprim (doses given at night)
  6 months–5 years 25 mg
  6 years–12 years 50 mg
  12+ years 100 mg
- cefadroxil 125 mg at night

dosage with impaired renal function

- antibiotics are commonly excreted by the kidneys but do not accumulate significantly with a creatinine clearance >30 ml/min
- with creatinine clearance <30 ml/min reduced dosage is required particularly with co-trimoxazole, and cefadroxil
- for gentamicin reduced dosage is required with creatinine clearance <70 ml/min

TREATMENT PLAN FOR SKIN INFECTIONS

- systemic antibiotics are preferable to local antibiotics to avoid skin sensitization
- crusts should be removed by bathing with water and/or Savlodil

cellulitis and erysipelas

- usually streptococcal

for adult

- phenoxymethylpenicillin
  500 mg six hourly orally
- benzylpenicillin 600 mg six hourly i.m. in ill patients
- erythromycin if *penicillin sensitive*
  500 mg six hourly

(*note*: slow resolution and may require 7–14 days treatment)

impetigo

- usually staphylococcal (may be penicillinase-producing) or streptococcal

for adult

- flucloxacillin
  500 mg six hourly, *or*
  erythromycin
  500 mg six hourly

for children

- flucloxacillin
  (doses six hourly)
  1–7 years 125 mg
  7+ years 250 mg
- erythromycin if *penicillin sensitive* (doses six hourly)
  0–1 years 62.5 mg
  1–5 years 125 mg
  6–12 years 250 mg

boils or abscesses

- usually staphylococcal
- flucloxacillin 500 mg
  six hourly
- erythromycin 600 mg
  six hourly

TREATMENT PLAN FOR CANDIDIASIS

Note: look for possible cause such as diabetes

oral candidiasis

for adult

- nystatin tablets (500 000 units)
  sucked six hourly (taste nasty) *or*
- nystatin pastilles (100 000 units)
  sucked six hourly (pleasanter taste if you like aniseed) *or*
- amphotericin lozenges
  one sucked six hourly for 1 week
- *note*: dentures should be removed and soaked in sodium
  hypochlorite solution

for children

- miconazole oral gel
  (apply gel around mouth and treat for 1 week)
  under 2 years 2.5 ml 12 hourly
  2–6 years 5 ml 12 hourly
  over 6 years 5 ml six hourly

vaginal candidiasis

- nystatin pessaries (100 000 units)
  for 14 nights, *or*
- clotrimazole vaginal tablets
  100 mg for six nights *or*
  200 mg for three nights *or*
  500 mg as single dose

13 DIABETES

WHAT IS IT?

- **diabetes** is not a single disease but a state of permanently disordered carbohydrate metabolism from a relative or absolute deficiency of insulin

- diabetes is **diagnosed** by raised blood sugar levels:
    fasting blood sugar >8 mmol/l
    random or after glucose load
        >11 mmol/l

- **two clinical types**

type 1

- there is a near **absolute** deficiency of insulin production

- insulin replacement is essential for maintenance of health and prevention of disease through normal blood sugar control

type 2

- there is a **relative** deficiency of insulin through insufficient production by the pancreas or inefficient utilization in the body

- the principles of treatment are diet to reduce intake of foods requiring insulin for metabolism and drugs to stimulate extra insulin production

WHO GETS IT WHEN?

- overall **age incidence** of diabetes increases with age

- **type 1 diabetes** occurs more frequently in young persons but can occur at any age

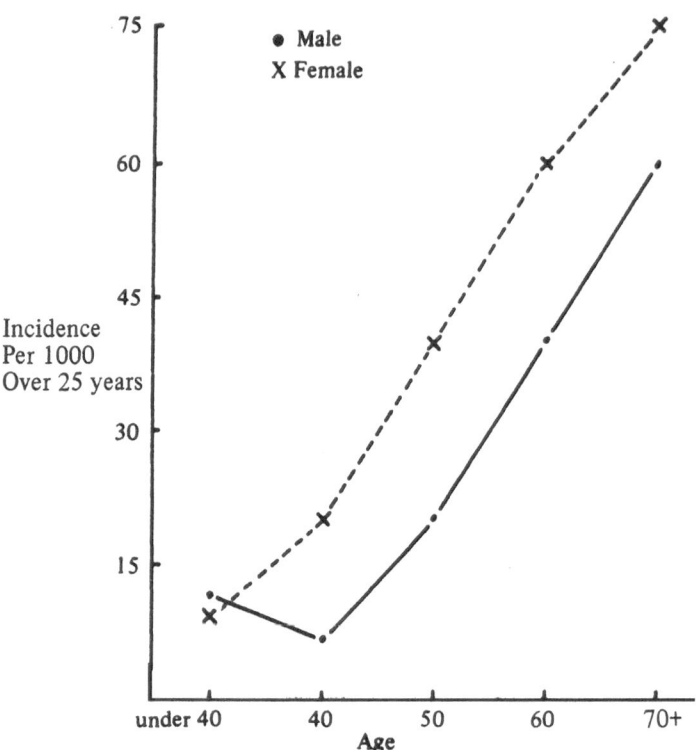

Incidence
Per 1000
Over 25 years

Age

- Male
X Female

Diabetes in a general practice with 2500 persons (annual numbers)		
New cases diagnoses		3
Known diabetics		
Type 1 on insulin	10	
Type 2 on diet	5	
on drugs	10	25
Possible undiagnosed diabetics in the practice		25

- **type 2 diabetes** occurs more often in middle and old age and is termed 'mature onset'

- there are more type 2 diabetics than type 1

WHAT HAPPENS?

- diabetes shortens life expectancy by one-third

- diabetics have higher mortality from:
  ischaemic heart disease and other
  cardiovascular disorders
  kidney disease and failure
  infections

ketoacidosis
diabetes being a risk factor in many
general diseases

- mortality and morbidity are reduced by
good control

- most diabetics do NOT develop **serious
complications** and when they do occur,
they are related to the duration of the
disease and to less than good control

complications

- rates in diabetics of over 10 years
standing:

Eyes	
retinopathy	15%
blind	8%
Heart	
IHD: cause of death in diabetics	50%
(in non-diabetics)	(25%)
Peripheral vascular disease	
intermittent claudication	3%
gangrene	1%
Kidneys	
diabetic glomerulosclerosis	10%[a]
Neuropathy	5%

([a] hospital cases)

DIABETES: RECAP

- known diabetes affects 1% of
population

- two types:
  type 1 requiring insulin
  replacement
  type 2 controlled by diet and
  drugs

- diabetics have a reduced life
expectancy and are prone to
complications

- complications are related to
duration of the disease and to
effectiveness of control

WHAT TREATMENT?

> **objectives**
> - control of hyperglycaemia
> - prolongation of life
> - prevention of complications
> - relief of symptoms
> - maintenance of normal quality of life
> - early diagnosis

DRUGS: ORAL HYPOGLYCAEMICS

SULPHONYLUREAS

what are they and how do they work?
- increase the release of endogenous insulin and augment its peripheral effects

effects

benefits
- control of type II (non-ketotic) diabetes when not controlled by diet

risks
- weight gain if diet not controlled
- hypoglycaemia (particularly chlorpropamide) if dose too high or patient fasts
- tolbutamide or chlorpropamide can cause fluid retention, therefore avoid in cardiac failure
- nausea, vomiting, rashes and drug fever
- flushing with alcohol (chlorpropamide only)

interactions
- effects enhanced by aspirin, sulphanamides, anticoagulants
- symptoms of hypoglycaemia masked by β-blockers

what available?

tolbutamide	– cheap, short-acting and effective
chlorpropamide	– long-acting, adverse effects common
glibenclamide	– effective and moderately long-acting
glipizide	– short-acting

which to use?

- tolbutamide or glibenclamide

- glipizide, when serious renal involvement

how to use?

- must be combined with diet, otherwise high risk of considerable weight gain

- **tolbutamide**
  day 1 3 g (six tablets)
  day 2 2 g (four tablets)
  day 3 1 g (two tablets)
  then adjust as necessary
  can be taken as single morning dose
  or in divided doses

- **glibenclamide**
  5 mg daily with breakfast (elderly 2.5 mg)
  (maximum 15 mg daily)

- **note**: type II diabetics may develop ketotic crisis precipitated by infections etc. and require insulin temporarily

BIGUANIDES: METFORMIN

what is it and how does it work?

- decreases glucose absorption from gut and increases its uptake into the tissues

effects

benefits

- controls blood glucose in type II diabetics

- can be combined with sulphonylureas
- reduces appetite and may make weight control easier

risks
- do NOT use in renal or liver disease, in alcoholism and severe infections
- slight risk of lactic acidosis
- nausea and gut upsets

how to use? metformin 500 mg eight hourly with food (maximum 3 g daily)

INSULINS

what are they and how do they work?
- polypeptides which promote glucose uptake by tissues
- increase glycogen formation
- promote synthesis of protein and prevent fat breakdown

effects

benefits
- control type I (ketotic) diabetes
- also used for other types of diabetes which are out of control
- used to control diabetes in pregnancy, major surgery and severe illness

risks
- hypoglycaemia if balance between insulin dosage and diet is incorrect
- ketoacidosis if insulin treatment is inadequate or is due to complicating factors (e.g. infections)
- allergic reactions (redness and itching) at injection sites
- fat atrophy at injection sites
- insulin resistance (more than 200 units daily) is rare

what available?

• a very large number of insulins now
available – classified by:

> *origin*
>
> • animal – bovine
>   porcine
>
> • human
>
> *purity*
>
> • human monocomponent, very
>   low immunogenicity
>
> • animal – monocomponent, low
>   immunogenicity
>   impure, immunogenic
>
> *duration of action*
>
> • short (neutral, soluble) $\frac{1}{2}$–6 h
>
> • intermediate (isophane insulins,
>   amorphous preparations) 4–14 h
>
> • long (insulin zinc suspensions or
>   crystalline preparations) 12–30 h
>
> • in addition *bisphasic insulins*
>   (mixture) have 2 peaks of activity
>   over   2–10 h

**human insulins and
monocomponent porcine
insulin**

• these are very similar and are
recommended for:
    diabetics first starting on insulin
    pregnant diabetics (insulin antibodies
        cross placenta)
    diabetics with
        allergies to insulin
        fat atrophy
        insulin resistance

• several options are available
    short-acting Human Actrapid
        (porcine equivalent – Actrapid MC)
    intermediate-acting Human Monotard
        (amorphous + crystalline
        (porcine equivalent – Monotard MC)

long-acting Human Ultratard (crystalline)
(equivalent – Lentard MC)
biphasic Human Mixtard
(neutral + isophane)
(porcine equivalent – Mixtard 30/70)

bovine insulins

- recommended for diabetics already satisfactorily stabilized on this type of insulin

short-acting	Neusulin
intermediate-acting	Neuphane
long-acting	Neulente

- note: Many other similar insulins available which are as satisfactory

points on administration of insulin

- insulin is given subcutaneously – 100 units/ml strength is now used with special graduated syringe

- sites for injection should be rotated; the rate of absorption is more rapid from the abdomen than from limbs, and is slowed by decreased blood flow, i.e. cold, shock

- spirit should not be used to clean the skin as it can cause hardening

- if soluble insulin is mixed with other insulins (particularly zinc suspension) the absorption of soluble insulin is slowed

- some reduction of dose (10–20%) is required on changing from bovine to porcine or human insulin

- during illness insulin requirements are usually increased

TREATMENT PLAN

note:
- make sure diagnosis is accurate (exclude low renal threshold) because treatment is for life

general measures
- each diabetic is an individual and management has to be personalized and flexible
- management should be well organized and easily understood and followed by all concerned, i.e. diabetic, family, GP team and hospital
- management involves:
  self care
  GP care possibly at a clinic or some other plan with regular checks on blood sugar, weight, vision and health
  hospital care at diabetic unit
  shared care involving all
- aims should be:
  type I to maintain normoglycaemia
  type II to control symptoms and keep urine free of sugar

diet
- essential for all diabetics to achieve ideal weight
- reduce total (and especially saturated) fats
- reduce carbohydrate intake and eat as 'slow release' foods such as vegetables
- reduce total calories to match activity needs
- increase fibre foods

mature onset – mild (typo II)
- diet alone may achieve normoglycaemia
  if not controlled within a month, *then*
- glibenclamide 2.5–15 mg daily
  (raise dose cautiously and slowly especially in elderly)

if this fails
- metformin 500 mg–1 g daily
  (in combination with glibenclamide)
- PATIENT MUST BE SEEN REGULARLY
- A REGISTER OF DIABETIC PATIENTS SHOULD BE KEPT

young onset – severe (type I)

- insulin replacement necessary
- basic plan should be to commence with neutral (soluble pH adjusted) insulin e.g. Actrapid MC, *or* biphasic e.g. Mixtard
- individual adjustments as required
- PATIENT MUST BE SEEN REGULARLY AT HOSPITAL AND/OR IN GENERAL PRACTICE FOR ASSESSMENT

complicated diabetes

- *children*: insulin necessary with special provisions for growth
- *elderly*: more important to avoid hypoglycaemia than to try to achieve normoglycaemia
- *pregnancy*: supervision at special unit to achieve as absolute normoglycaemia as possible – change to human or monocomponent insulin
- *complications*: early diagnosis and treatment – of retinopathy, glomerulosclerosis, peripheral vascular disease and neuropathy – are necessary to try and prevent progressive deterioration

14   **PSYCHIATRIC DISORDERS**

WHAT ARE THEY?

- although psychiatric disorders are prevalent in all clinical fields, they present particular problems of accurate and substantiated diagnosis and definition

- this is because they are largely based on symptoms and other subjective evidence

- the most frequent diagnoses are:
  anxiety
  depression
  insomnia
  personal and personality problems
  psychosomatic disorders
  psychosis and brain failure (dementias)
  others – including alcoholism, effects of drugs

- the nature of the common psychiatric disorders is uncertain in terms of biochemical and other changes

WHO GETS THEM WHEN?

- although they occur at all ages and affect both sexes they tend to be more prevalent in women and in early adult and middle-age

- about 15–20% of all consultations in British general practice are for diagnosed psychiatric disorders

- another sizeable proportion of the population is suffering from emotional problems and do not consult their doctor

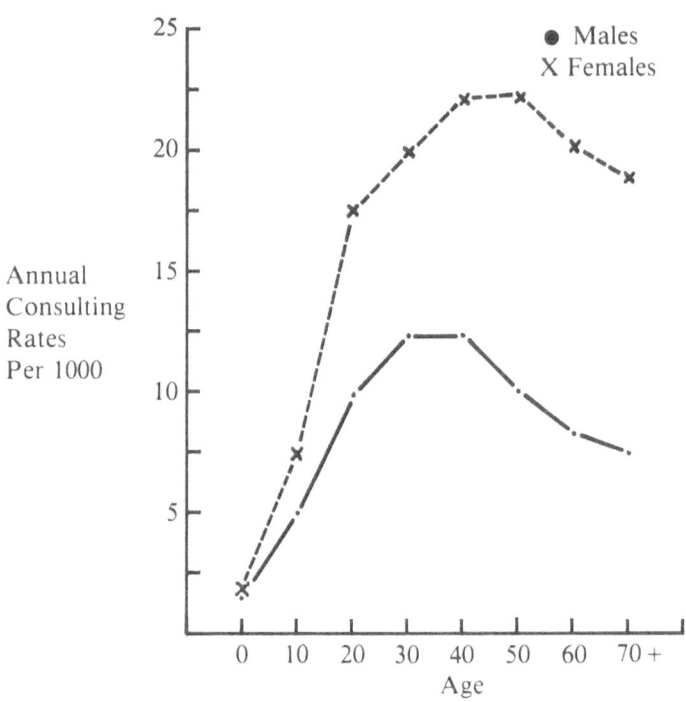

- **annual prevalence** of psychiatric problems in a general practice of 2500

Persons consulting	375
Referred to psychiatrist	20
Parasuicide	1
Suicide	1 in 5 years

WHAT HAPPENS?

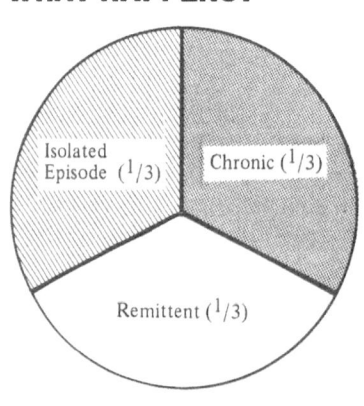

- with such highly individual conditions and situations the course and outcome may be difficult to predict

- in general terms the outcomes tend to be:
  one third suffer an **isolated single episode**
  one third suffer **intermittent attacks** related to exogenous or endogenous factors
  one third become **chronic**

PSYCHIATRIC DISORDERS

PSYCHIATRIC DISORDERS: A RECAP

- frequent (15% of all consultations in general practice)
- nature and causes uncertain
- diagnosis and classification imprecise
- 'Three thirds' pattern of natural history with a sizeable proportion of 'chronic' cases

WHAT TREATMENT?

objectives

- to promote self-help and family support and understanding
- to prevent – where there are preventable factors
- to define 'at-risk' individuals for special care and help
- to provide/organize treatment and assistance

DRUGS

ANTIDEPRESSANTS

what are they and how do they work?

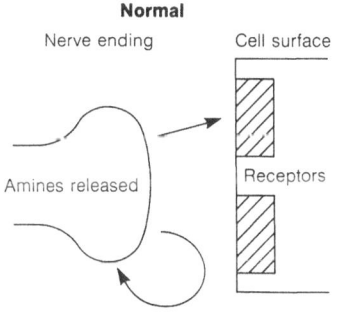

Normal

Nerve ending   Cell surface

Amines released

Receptors

Re-uptake of amine

- all the current antidepressant drugs probably produce their therapeutic effects by raising the concentrations of brain amines

tricyclics

- imipramine
- amitriptyline

tricyclic – anxiolytics

- dothiepin
- doxepin

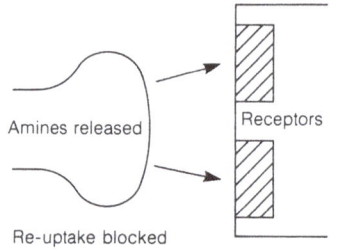

After Tricyclic Anti-depressant

Amines released

Receptors

Re-uptake blocked

tetracyclics and others

- mianserin
- trazodone

monoamine oxidase inhibitors (MAOIs)

- phenelzine

tricyclics

effects

benefits

- relief of depression in about 80% of those treated
- *note*: response is slow –
  sleep disturbance corrected quickly, but the depressive symptoms may take up to 4 weeks to show any evidence of improvement

risks

- anticholinergic effects (do NOT use in glaucoma or with prostatic symptoms)
- dry mouth and constipation which may be worrying and troublesome
- cardiac arrhythmias may cause sudden death
- hypotension (in elderly)

interactions

- interaction with adrenaline e.g. in local anaesthetics (dental) causing hypertensive crisis
- enhances effects of alcohol
- do not combine well with MAOIs

| **which to use?** | • imipramine or amitriptyline are satisfactory, but side effects are common |
| | • amitriptyline has more sedative actions |

how to use?

imipramine/amitriptyline	• single dose of 50–75 mg (elderly 25 mg) at night may be increased to 100–150 mg
	• warn of possible adverse effects
	• stress delay in achieving beneficial response
	• treatment should be continued for 6–9 months and then reduce dose slowly to avoid withdrawal symptoms
	• in some patients may need to be continued for some years

tricyclic – anxiolytics

effects

| *benefits* | • less powerful antidepressant actions but relieve associated anxiety |
| | • less cardiotoxic |

| *risks* | • as with tricyclics |

how to use?

| *dothiepin* | • single dose at night of 75 mg and increasing to 150 mg if necessary |

| *doxepin* | • single dose at night of 25–50 mg and increasing to 300 mg if necessary |

tetracyclics and others

effects

benefits
- relief of depression
- less dangerous with overdose
- no anticholinergic and no cardiotoxic effects

risks
- mianserin – some doubts on efficacy
- marked sedative effects with mianserin and may cause blood dyscrasias, liver damage and arthritis
- trazodone causes drowsiness and is expensive

which to use?
- these are *not* first line antidepressants
- should be considered only if tricyclics are contraindicated

monoamine-oxidase inhibitors (MAOIs)

what are they and how do they work?
- inhibit breakdown of amines in the brain (and elsewhere too)

effects

benefits
- relief of depression in 1–3 weeks
- particularly effective in neurotic depression

risks
- many
- exaggerate effects of amines in food and drugs and may rarely produce a hypertensive crisis (*note*: beware the MAOI patient who develops a severe headache)

- **foods** with amines are:
    cheeses, wines, beers, broadbean pods,
    yeast extracts, bananas and pickled
    herrings

- **drugs** with amines are:
    'cold cures' with vasoconstrictors,
    levodopa and tricyclic antidepressants

- antidote is phentolamine 5–10 mg i.v. and
    repeated if necessary

- may cause drowsiness, agitation,
    hypotension and liver damage

interactions

- interact with centrally acting drugs,
    particularly pethidine

how to use?

- explain risks to patient and why it should
    be used

- **phenelzine**:
    15 mg three times daily
    increase to four times daily after 2 weeks
        if necessary

lithium

what is it and how does it work?

- lithium is an element, generally used as
    the carbonate

- mode of action unknown

effects

benefits

- beneficial in the prevention of mood
    swings in manic-depressives and in
    relieving manic attacks

risks

- many are **dose-related**
    tremor
    diarrhoea, thirst
    ataxia
    confusion
    coma
    death

- **non-dose related**
  - thyroid function upsets
  - renal damage
- do NOT use in pregnancy, surgery, renal disorders, and disorders of sodium metabolism

interactions

- interactions with diuretics – leads to retention of lithium and toxic effects
- do NOT use with anti-psychotic drugs because extrapyramidal effects are increased

how to use?

- consult with psychiatrist before use
- before treatment check:
  plasma creatinine, thyroid function, ECG and blood picture
- repeat creatinine and thyroid function tests six monthly

lithium carbonate

- 400 mg in single dose at night
- check plasma lithium concentrations to achieve levels of 0.4–0.9 mmol/l
- tests should be weekly at first and then every few months
- test should be at least 12 h after last dose

HYPNOTICS AND ANXIOLYTICS
BENZODIAZEPINES

what are they and how do they work?

- group of drugs which potentiate the natural inhibitor GABA in the brain

effects

benefits

- produce sedation and sleep with minimal risk from overdose

- relax skeletal muscles
- some are anti-convulsant

risks
- dependence with prolonged use
- unpleasant withdrawal symptoms (3–8 days after stopping drug)
- in mild dependence
  insomnia
  anxiety
- in more severe dependence
  hallucinations
  depersonalization
  perceptual disorders
  fits
  (may persist for several weeks)
- impaired physical and mental efficiency
- rarely disinhibition with aggressive behaviour

what to use?
- wide choice

hypnotics
triazolam (short-acting)
temazepam (short-acting)
diazepam (long-acting)
nitrazepam (long-acting)

anxiolytics
diazepam
lorazepam

anti-convulsants
diazepam
clonazepam

how to use?

insomnia
- triazolam: 0.125–0.25 mg at night (especially suitable for elderly)
- temazepam: 10–20 mg at night
- diazepam: 2.5–10 mg at night

- ideally, use for only 2 weeks but patients often seek longer treatment, when effectiveness diminishes and dependence develops

anxiety
- diazepam: 2–5 mg three times daily or 5 mg at night
- lorazepam: 1–2.5 mg twice daily
- ideally, only use for short time but if relieved patients often ask for long-term

PSYCHOTROPIC DRUGS
PHENOTHIAZINES AND BUTYROPHENONES

what are they and how do they work?
- large group
- dopamine antagonists in the brain, also with anticholinergic and adrenergic blocking actions

effects

benefits
- antipsychotic
- antihallucinatory
- sedative
- anti-emetic and suppress hiccough

risks
- extrapyramidal effects with acute dystonia, parkinsonism, restlessness (akasthesia)
- tardive dyskinesia – in 15% on long-term therapy (may not recover on stopping drug)
- cholestatic jaundice (in 4% on chlorpromazine)
- anticholinergic effects (dry mouth, urinary retention and constipation)
- hypotension (postural)
- rashes

PSYCHIATRIC DISORDERS

- hyperpyrexia (malignant syndrome)
- do NOT use where glaucoma, prostatism, epilepsy and alcohol withdrawal as may cause fits

what available and how to use?
- variety of opinions

acute confusional states
- chlorpromazine 50–200 mg orally
  25–50 mg i.m.

elderly confusional states
- treat any precipitating cause
- thioridazine 25–50 mg single dose at night
  30–100 mg in a day
- promazine 50 mg three times daily

long-term management of schizophrenia

oral
- chlorpromazine 100–1000 mg daily in divided doses
- promazine (in elderly) 75–400 mg daily in divided doses
- haloperidol 5–40 mg daily in divided doses
- pimozide 2–16 mg single daily dose

Drug	Sedation	Extra-pyramidal effects	Usage
Chlorprom-azine	+ +	+ +	acute and long-term
Promazine	I	+ +	acute and long-term
Haloperidol	+	+ + +	acute, sometimes long-term
Pimozide	+	(+)	long-term only

depot preparations

- aid compliance, but effects are variable due to individual differences in mobilization and metabolism
- fluphenazine decanoate 12.5–50 mg i.m. (repeated at 2–4 week intervals)

TREATMENT PLAN

note:

- a precise aetiological and biochemical based diagnosis is not possible
- a pragmatic approach has to be accepted
- often a diagnostic label leads to use of certain drugs
- sometimes an available drug may lead to application of a diagnostic label

general measures

- more than anything else flexible personal care, support and understanding are necessary for the patient and family
- the general practitioner is in a particularly good situation over the years to come to know patients and families and their psychoses and environments and the nature and outcomes of their disorders
- in many situations a non-medication 'psychotherapy' is most important, but this must be tailored and modified to individual doctors and individual patients
- the great majority of psychiatric disorders are diagnosed and managed by GPs and few are referred to psychiatrists: most referrals are psychotics, severe depressions, phobic anxiety states and some personality disorders
- *drugs* (when indicated)

anxiety states

- the 'anxiety' may be in the patient but the anxious patient often creates an 'anxiety response' in the doctor who is consulted
- the first measures must be to provide a sympathetic response to the patient's anxieties, to understand and to allay them through listening, explanation and support
- there are *short-term anxiety states* that require short term measures where simple psychotherapy is the more important and where drugs can be given safely for a short time
- there are *long-term chronic anxiety states* usually coupled with insoluble personality and environmental problems – regular long-term supportive consultations are necessary but drugs are much more likely to be prescribed; these have largely a placebo effect but there are special risks of developing dependency

- *drugs* do help in relieving tensions, they do sedate but can create dependency with unpleasant withdrawal features
- drugs should be given
    for short limited periods
    in small supplies
- *particular care should be taken to avoid 'repeat prescriptions' for 'unseen patients'*
- appropriate daily anxiolytics are:
    diazepam 2–15 mg
    lorazepam 1–5 mg
- where somatic symptoms are part of the presentation then a β-blocker can be helpful:
    propranolol 40–120 mg daily

insomnia

- first, ensure that there really is a problem; many complain of not sleeping when their sleep pattern is normal; elderly persons often sleep more in the day and less at night
- suitable short-term hypnotics for situations such as travelling and for worriers over the day ahead:
    triazolam 0.125–0.025 mg (elderly 0.125 mg)
    temazepam 10–20 mg
    (elderly 5–10 mg) at night
- insomnia associated with anxiety, grief and stress is best managed by supportive discussion but short-term hypnotic may be needed (for up to 2 weeks)
    triazolam 0.125–0.25 mg (elderly start with 0.125 mg)
    temazepam 10–20 mg
    (elderly 5–10 mg) at night, *or*
    diazepam 5–10 mg
    (elderly 2.5–10 mg) at night
- long-term insomnia is often due to underlying causes and may be difficult to manage; look out for:
    depression
    pain
    urinary frequency
    constipation
    heart failure
    dementia
- possible simple measures to assist sleep in long-term insomnia:
    quiet evening
    avoid late coffee/tea
    pre-bed exercise

PSYCHIATRIC DISORDERS

nightcap of alcohol will help to 'get off' to sleep but with tendency to early waking and dependence

- if unsuccessful, then either try to get patient to accept the situation, *or*
    antidepressant such as amitriptyline 50–75 mg at night

- benzodiazepines should be used only intermittently to cover difficult periods and not for long term

- in the elderly avoid hypnotics if possible – try and achieve acceptance that poor sleep is normal

- if hypnotic is to be used in elderly:
    triazolam 0.125–0.25 mg at night is short-acting with little hangover effect
    temazepam 5–10 mg at night but it is short acting and early waking may occur
    nitrazepam 5–10 mg at night but there is often a 'hang-over' next day

- if night confusion is a problem in the elderly:
    thioridazine 25–50 mg at night

stopping benzodiazepines

- withdrawal symptoms develop within 4 days – they will be more severe with short-acting benzodiazepines

- withdrawal should be step-by-step over at least a month, for example:
    diazepam by 2 mg daily at each step
    lorazepam by 0.5 mg daily at each step
    nitrazepam by 5 mg daily at each step
    temazepam by 5 mg daily at each step
    triazolam by 0.125 mg daily at each step

- the speed of withdrawal should be regulated by patient's symptoms

- occasionally depression will occur during withdrawal and antidepressants will help

- the patient should be seen at least once weekly for assessment and support

depression

- 'depression' may be a difficult diagnosis

- as the nature and causation are uncertain so management has to be pragmatic

- wide clinical range of presentations from minor depressions with anxiety and other neurotic symptoms through to severe psychotic depressions which may be life threatening

- the course of the illness is unpredictable and the responses to antidepressant drugs are uncertain

- the choice and selection of antidepressants rest on the doctor's own interpretation and understanding of his patient and of his familiarity with the drug

as a general guide:

- for less severe depression with anxiety features
  amitriptyline 50–150 mg daily with all or most of the dose at night, or
  dothiepin 75–150 mg daily with all or most of the dose at night

- for more severe depression with retardation
  imipramine 75–150 mg daily in divided doses or at night

- inform patients that it will take up to four weeks for improvement to be noticeable, mention possible side effects and that medication may be required for months and occasionally for years

psychoses

- best managed in collaboraton with the local psychiatric service

- general practitioner is involved in the earliest stages which may be dramatic and in long-term care which may be trying

acute confusional states and mania

- chlorpromazine 25–50 mg i.m.
  repeated in 6–8 h if necessary
  50–200 mg daily orally

long-term control of schizophrenia

- chlorpromazine 100–800 mg daily
  in divided doses, or

- haloperidol 5–40 mg daily
  in divided doses, or

- by depot preparations as
  fluphenazine 12.5 mg–25 mg i.m.
  every 2–4 weeks

- note: high risk of development of extrapyramidal symptoms and drowsiness

prevention of manic-depression

- lithium carbonate 400 mg daily

- note: a narrow therapeutic/toxic ratio therefore monitor plasma lithium levels regularly (therapeutic range 0.4–0.9 mmol/l)

15   TERMINAL CARE

WHAT IS IT?

- 'terminal care' is the management of the extended process of dying

- **dying** takes various forms and is of varying durations: at one end of the spectrum it is sudden and unexpected and at the other end it is a long-drawn-out process ending in 'a happy release'

- **terminal care** is much more than 'cancer care' – it is personal and family care for patients dying from any cause of any duration and it must be sensitive, human and humane care

- **terminal care** is much more concerned with **comfort** of the dying and the family and with **relief** of symptoms than with heroic efforts at care

- one important part of such care is the avoidance of well-meaning but futile therapies that cause unnecessary suffering

WHO DIES FROM WHAT AND WHERE?

causes of death

- in Britain there are around 600 000 deaths per year (or 11 per 1000 of the population)

- the **major causes of death in UK** are:

	%
Ischaemic heart disease (IHD)	25
Cancers	23
Bronchitis and pneumonia	13
Strokes	12
Accidents	3
Others	24
	100

where?

- 2/3 of deaths now take place in hospitals
- 1/5 at home
- 1/20 in hospices
- 1/10 'elsewhere' (in public places etc.)

frequency of need

- **terminal care** involves probably no more than 1 in 3 of all deaths

numbers of deaths

- in a general practice of 2500 persons the annual numbers of deaths will be:

Cause	Numbers
IHD	5
Cancers	5
Bronchitis and pneumonia	3
Strokes	3
Others	9
	25

- of these only four or five will be cared for terminally at home

WHAT HAPPENS?

- estimations of life expectancies ('how long has he got to live?') by doctors are fraught with imprecision
- a figure may be sought but forecasting may be distressing if wrong
- the problems and challenges in terminal care depend on the cause, the course and the individual
- **death is a once-in-a-lifetime experience for everyone**

problems to manage? the most prominent problems to be managed in terminal care are:

> - fear, bewilderment and uncertainty
> - anxiety over one's suffering and one's behaviour
> - depression and dejection
> - pain and discomfort
> - sleeplessness
> - breathlessness
> - constipation
> - diarrhoea
> - incontinence
> - loss of appetite
> - nausea and vomiting
> - bed sores

TERMINAL CARE: RECAP
- the mortality of life is 100%
- dying is a once in-a-lifetime experience
- 'terminal care' of extended dying involves a minority of deaths, many are quick and unexpected
- conditions requiring terminal care will be
  cancers
  progressive heart failure
  strokes and other neurological diseases
  chronic respiratory failure
  dementias
- problems in terminal care will relate to the individual

WHAT TREATMENT?

Objectives
- total humane care of the patient and the family
- good personal communication, rapport, support and comfort
- symptom relief that should be preventive and anticipatory as well as specific
- care by a caring team but not so large as to make communication and rapport difficult

DRUGS WITH PARTICULAR REFERENCE TO PAIN RELIEF

General rules in use of analgesics in terminal care
- give regularly to prevent pain and not only when pain occurs
- give in sufficient dosage to keep patient free of pain all the time
- give orally whenever possible for smoother pain control

SIMPLE ANALGESICS

what are they and how do they work?

aspirin
- cyclo-oxygenase inhibitor
- anti-inflammatory

paracetamol
- mild central analgesic

combinations with a weak opiate	• co-codaprin: aspirin 400 mg + codeine 8 mg
	• co-proxamol: paracetamol 325 mg + dextropropoxyphene 32.5 mg (additional opiate may enhance analgesic effects)

effects

benefits	• relief in mild–moderate pain for 4–6 h
	• aspirin and other NSAIAs are especially effective in secondary bone deposits
risks	• aspirin (see p. 9)
	• paracetamol – hepatotoxic in overdose
	• co-codaprin and co-proxamol – constipation and dizziness
	• overdose of co-proxamol may cause respiratory depression and circulatory collapse, potentiated by alcohol

how to use?

	• patient responses are variable and trial and error approach is appropriate
	• commence with single drug but can be used in combinations with strong analgesics if pain not controlled
paracetamol	• **adult** 1 g every 4–6 h
	• **child** (age 1–5) 120–250 mg every 4–6 h
	• **child** (age 6–12) 250–500 mg every 4–6 h
aspirin (dispersible)	• **adult** 600 mg every 4–6 h
	• **child** (do not use in under 12s) 300 mg every 4–6 h
co-codaprin	• one or two tablets every 4–6 h

co-proxamol • one or two tablets every 6 h

OPIATES

what are they and how do • morphine and **diamorphine**
they work? (diamorphine is converted into morphine
in the body)

Site of action of opioids • stimulate opiate receptors in the brain and
spinal cord which inhibit pain sensation

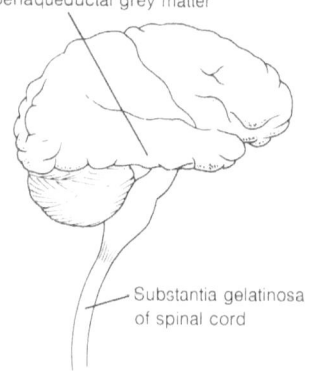

On thalamus and
periaqueductal grey matter

Substantia gelatinosa
of spinal cord

effects

benefits • relief of pain for 4–6 h in adequate dosage

• sedative and euphoriant actions

• suppress cough

risks • constipation, virtually in all cases,
therefore regular laxatives are helpful

• nausea/vomiting, in about one-third, but
then may cease in a few days
(give prochlorperazine 12.5 mg, i.m., or
10 mg oral and then eight hourly, or
haloperidol 3 mg twelve hourly)

• nightmares and hallucinations, rarely, can
be controlled by lowering dose

• dependence – this is not important in
terminal care

• respiratory depression, usually only a
problem with large overdosage

188

how to use?

for persistent pain

- **diamorphine** as elixir
  commence with 10 mg in 10 ml four hourly
  (half dose in elderly) and review after a
  day or two and then increase dosage
  and/or frequency as necessary to prevent
  pain.

- **slow release morphine** (SR-MST) may be
  substituted – effective in a twice daily dose

- **note**: 20 mg of diamorphine every 4 h is
  equivalent to 60 mg of morphine SR every
  12 h

- injections of opiates are rarely necessary
  in management of pain in terminal illness

OTHER OPIATES FOR SPECIAL INDICATIONS

dextromoramide

- short and quick action for particularly
  painful episodes

- 5–15 mg orally or sublingual

Diconal (dipipanone and cyclizine, an antiemetic)

- may be too sedating

- one or two tablets by mouth

Oxycodone

- as a suppository (30 mg)

- useful as an overnight analgesic

PARTIAL AGONISTS

what are they and how do they work?

- combined stimulation and blocking
  effects on opioid receptors – these result
  in a powerful analgesic effect with less risk
  of dependence

- buprenorphine is most widely used

- large first-pass action so given
  sublingually

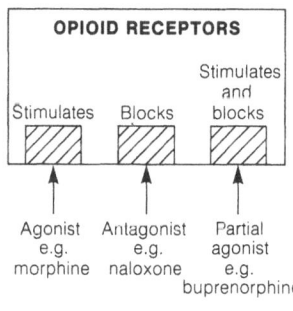

effects

benefits
- relief of moderate–severe pain for 6–8 h
- less constipating and less respiratory depression than morphine

risks
- nausea/vomiting (may need withdrawal)
- other adverse effects less marked than morphine
- toxicity requires larger doses of naloxone for reversal than for morphine

how to use?
- buprenorphine tablets 200µg sublingually every 6–8 h
- buprenorphine injection 300 µg i.m. every 6–8 h
- *note:* because of partial blockade of opioid receptors by buprenorphine the effect of high doses of morphine given concurrently is reduced – this does not apply in the usual therapeutic range

PAIN RELIEF WITHOUT DRUGS
relief of pain can also be achieved in other ways as by radiotherapy and nerve blocks

TREATMENT PLAN

note:

- only about 1/3 of deaths involve extended terminal care
- the same principles of caring for the dying apply everywhere – in hospitals, homes and hospices

general measures

- of greatest value and importance is a relaxed, quiet and hopeful approach by the carers
- care of the dying involves a team of nurses, doctors, family and friends
- comfort and relief rather than heroic attempts at cure
- above all human concern, kindness, understanding and regular contact and communication

pain

Aim: a graded and flexible approach for each person to control pain by anticipation and taking the medication *before* it occurs, requiring regular medication

mild

- aspirin 600–900 mg every few hours, *or*
- paracetamol 0.5–1.0 g every few hours, *or*
- co-proxamol every few hours

moderate–severe

- opiates are most effective in controlling moderate–severe pain
- in terminal care the concern is to control pain and not to worry about creating possible addiction
- morphine or diamorphine:
  commence with diamorphine elixir 5–10 mg every 4 h, assess effectiveness frequently and increase dosage until painfree. A change can then be made to morphine SR tablets 6–12 hourly (ratio of diamorphine to morphine SR is 1:1) If oral route is not possible then use subcutaneous diamorphine (ratio oral to s.c. is 2:1) four hourly or use oxycodone suppositories 30 mg every 8 h
- inevitably constipation ensues and laxatives should be prescribed prophylactically
- bone pain from secondary deposits may be relieved by indomethacin 25–50 mg three times daily by mouth

- pain may be caused by causes amenable to radiotherapy and nerve blocks

nausea/vomiting

- may be due to either opiates or the disease
- chlorpromazine 25–50 mg every 4–8 h, *or* haloperidol 500 μg to 3 mg twice daily (less sedating)
- prednisolone 10 mg twice daily may improve appetite and wellbeing and make pain control easier

cough

- if no remediable cause, such as infection, then relief by:
  diamorphine linctus, *or*
  methadone linctus

constipation

- Senokot with if necessary docusate sodium *or*
  suppositories of glycerine or bisacodyl, *or*
  enema

diarrhoea

- codeine phosphate 30–60 mg every 8–12 h

INDEX